Journey To New Beginnings

Finding Peace Within

Debbie Ziemann, RN

Bloomington, IN  Milton Keynes, UK

authorHOUSE®

AuthorHouse™
1663 Liberty Drive, Suite 200
Bloomington, IN 47403
www.authorhouse.com
Phone: 1-800-839-8640

AuthorHouse™ UK Ltd.
500 Avebury Boulevard
Central Milton Keynes, MK9 2BE
www.authorhouse.co.uk
Phone: 08001974150

This book is a work of non-fiction. Unless otherwise noted, the author and the publisher make no explicit guarantees as to the accuracy of the information contained in this book and in some cases, names of people and places have been altered to protect their privacy.

First published by AuthorHouse 4/26/2007

ISBN: 978-1-4259-7771-9 (e)
ISBN: 978-1-4259-7769-6 (sc)
ISBN: 978-1-4259-7770-2 (hc)

Library of Congress Control Number: 2006909978
Printed in the United States of America
Bloomington, Indiana

This book is printed on acid-free paper.

Michael Josephson's What Will Matter is used with permission of the Josephson Instittute of Ethics. © 2007 Michael Josephson, one of the nation's leading ethicists, is the founder of the nonprofit, nonsectarian Josephson Institute of Ethics and the premier youth character education program, CHARACTER COUNTS! For more information or to make a donation, please visit www.charactercounts.org

I want to thank Angela McGerr, author of 'an Angel for every day', published by Quadrilee 2005 and Richard Rockwood who completed the illustrations, for allowing me to use Tual, on the cover of the book. Their image of this Angel was exactly what I had invisioned. an Angel for every day has helped me continue to use the power of the Universe as I continue on this journey and healing.

*The best way to celebrate life
is to share
your own unique self
with the world.*

Dedication

I dedicate this book to my mother, who passed away at the young age of fifty-four. She fought for twenty-two years, living her life with ovarian, bone and lung cancer. Her strength and courage, taking one day at a time, has given me the determination to be a breast cancer survivor. Her spirit has come to sit beside me in some of my most darkest moments, holding my hand and encouraging me to be strong and to survive.

I also dedicate this to my father, who recently passed away from bone cancer. Although we did not have the father–daughter relationship that I always wanted, he was still my father, and I loved him very much.

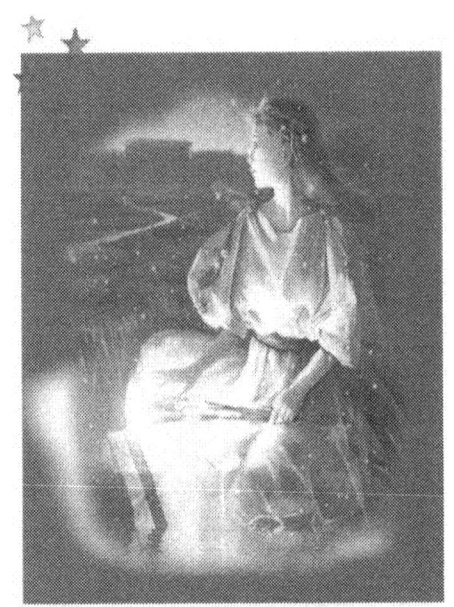

"My Personal Angel"

I often feel your presence
When I close my eyes at night,
I feel the gentle whisper of your wings
As you pass me by so light.

Your loving soul brings me comfort
As it did when you were here,
Drifting safely within reach
Letting me hold you dear.

Your heart helps to guide me
And your spirit calms my tears.
You give me the courage
I need to conquer my fears.
My thanks and my love
Go to my personal angel.
I take you with me every day
And of the things I do in life,
Your love and efforts I will repay.

I miss you.
Sandra J. Labadie, 2000

Introduction

The year following my breast cancer diagnosis, a total mastectomy, and completing chemotherapy, I felt as if I was out at sea in the midst of a storm. Darkness surrounded me and I was filled with despair. The faster I ran from the darkness, the closer it drew near. I became frightened, and soon learned that it was not going to be easy. I knew that the way to the light was to go directly into the darkness and face it, to learn, and then conquer my fear.

Anger soon started to consume me. I wasn't angry that I had breast cancer, but angry that it had happened in the second year of my marriage. I even found that after all the years of being estranged from my father, I was still angry. I became disillusioned with my presence within a company that no longer had compassion for their staff, and our employees were losing the ability to take care of patients and families that were going through the end-of-life process. Thus, I found myself deciding to resign and take some time off from the work force. I wanted to be able to make "happy memories" for my family. Health and family had become a priority, and there was nothing more important than family.

I also found that because of my inability to accept my new body image, I developed insecurities that would place my marriage in turmoil. We seldom found time for each other. My husband worked twelve-to-sixteen hours a day, six days a week, which started to make me feel that he did not want to be with me. Intimacy soon became a thing of the past, which lead to further insecurity. Because of my body's inability to respond to his touch, the frustration built until I thought I had lost control. We lost our desire and willingness to be close. It was not just I who was insecure. My husband was also becoming insecure, thinking that I didn't love him anymore because I didn't reach out to him physically. For awhile, we were like a four-legged table with a broken leg. We fought to make our marriage survive.

This book will share with you the turmoil that I experienced during the first year after I was diagnosed with breast cancer. I realized that having a mastectomy was far more devastating than I had realized in the beginning. My self-esteem and self-confidence had been destroyed, and I would need to learn how to re-establish myself so that I could go on with life and living. I will take you through the steps that I took to find my new self.

I looked for the person that I wanted to be, and to find. I found that I could find peace and comfort within myself by means of connecting with the Universe. The spiritual world. I could not rely on myself to heal, and I needed to allow God to take me in His hands and carry me. I learned to give myself to God, and allow him to handle the problems that I was not able to. I learned that my strength came from within, and from the energy of the Universe. Each of us has the choice to decide how we are going to react and respond. We have the choice to become a victim or fight to be a "Survivor."

I had to trust my desires and learn that I could make things happen. Maybe they did not happen when or as quickly as I wanted, but they happened. To my amazement, I learned that I could 'will' events to take place. I no longer believe that things happen by chance. They happen because we make them happen with positive thoughts and purpose.

Learning there is life after cancer, is one of the hardest journeys that I have been on in this life. My belief is that everything happens for a reason, and life is more real than ever before. We not only understand, but we also will celebrate when we understand. The celebration takes the form of caring more for people and friends, and building new and better relationships with family. I celebrate this new life by sharing my journey with others who are experiencing or have gone through this heartbreaking, devastating, and life-threatening ordeal.

As you start reading, I believe that you will feel the turmoil. I could not let some issues go. Those issues I state repeatedly because they weighed so heavily on my mind. Nevertheless, as I worked through this, fighting to allow myself the time to grieve, you will feel the peace that I started to feel within myself.

Cancer is so limited...
It cannot cripple Love,
It cannot shatter Hope,
It cannot corrode Faith,
It cannot eat away Peace.
It cannot destroy Confidence.
It cannot kill Friendship,
It cannot shut out Memories,
It cannot silence Courage,
It cannot invade the Soul,
It cannot reduce Eternal Life,
It cannot quench the Spirit,
And it cannot lessen the Power of the Resurrection!

-Author Unknown

Cancer begins with the word CAN. You can do anything that you want. You can be a survivor, when you learn that being a survivor is a state of mind that is dictated by you. No one else can teach you how to survive, not even your family, friends, and certainly not your co-workers. You have to find your own independent path that will lead you to finding yourself and what makes you happy. This new path will give you the sense of fulfillment, peace, and contentment, filling your life with compassion by sharing your love for life with others which brings the richness of living—the joy of being alive.

Everyone's path will be different and the speed in which we recover will vary. What may have worked for me, may not work for you. We cannot compare ourselves to others, and how they recovered. We have to remember that we are individuals with different personalities. We will take the path that is comfortable for each of us.

I hope that *Journey to New Beginnings* will provide you with a sense of comfort, and hope that there is life after breast cancer. Sharing my journey with you and others has helped me to heal. I will continue to grow and heal for the rest of my life. Each year will be another path to tread and to experience the joys of life and living. I will continue to allow my soul to flow with the energy from within, and without, breathing life and love into my world.

Gently With The Flow

If the sky above seems cloudy,
And you are left out in the rain,
If you are searching for a rainbow,
But the colors bring you pain,

If your world is not revolving,
And there is no end in sight,
If you are looking for the sunshine,
But all you see is night,

If all around are smiling,
But all you can do is frown,
If you are tired of all this living,
When life just brings you down,

Then look beyond your teardrops,
At the wonders of this land,
The beauty of a flower,
Like velvet in your hand.

Feel the sir sun around you,
The smell of new mown hay,
Laughing children in the park,
The innocence there at play.

Imagine floating with a butterfly,
As she flutters between the trees,
Or the whispers of the ocean,
In a hot summer's breeze.

Think of the taste of candy floss,
As it melts upon your tongue,
Or the melody of morning birds,
As they greet each day with song.

Remember words of beauty,
Told in your mother's embrace.
Feel the gentleness of her touch,
As she softly kissed your face.

Seek the good within you.
Cast the clouds from your sky.
Don't look toward the pavement,
But hold your head up high.

Think not what life owes you,
But of all you have to give.
Forget about tomorrow,
Then you can start to live.

So bless this age you are living in,
With the gifts you can bestow.
Don't disregard the stream of life,
Go gently with the flow.

-Author Unknown

Chapters

1. In The Midst of the Storm   1

2. In The Valley Is Where We Grow   53

3. Amazing New Paths Appear   61

4. Overwhelming Darkness Surrounds Me   69

5. Another Mountain   87

6. Discover The Limits of The Possible   101

7. Drawn By The Gentle Pull Of My Heart   114

8. Going Beyond Into The Impossible   119

9. The Universe Will Work In Unison With You   132

10. Walk Hand In Hand   138

11. Love Is Healing   141

12. Road To A New Beginning   147

13. Spiritual Path To Inner Peace   152

14. Food For Thought   156

What Will Matter

Ready or not,
someday it will call come to an end.
There will be no more sunrises,
no minutes, hours or days.

All the things you collected,
whether treasured or forgotten,
will pass to someone else.

Your wealth,
fame and temporal power
will shrivel to irrelevance.
It will not matter what you owned
or what you were owed.

So, too you hopes, ambitious, plan
And to-do lists will expire.
The wins and losses
That once seemed so important
Will fade away.

It won't matter where you came from,
Or on what side of the tracks you lived,
At the end.
It won't matter whether you were beautiful or
brilliant,
Even your gender and skin color will be irrelevant.

So what will matter?
How will the value of your days be measured?

What will matter is not what you bought,
but what you built,
not what you got,
but what you gave?

What will matter is not your success,
but your significance.

What will matter is not what you learned,
But what you taught.

What will matter is every act of integrity,
compassion,
courage or sacrifice that enriched,
Empowered or encouraged others to emulate your
example.

What will matter is not your competence,
But your character.
What will matter is not how many people you knew,
But how many will feel a lasting loss when you're
gone.

What will matter is not your memories,
but the memories that live in those who loved you.
What will matter is how long you will be
remembered,
by whom and for what.

Living a life that matters doesn't happen by
accident.
It's not a matter of circumstances but a choice.
Choose to live a life that matters.

Author Michael Josephson

Chapter One

In The Midst of the Storm

*Much of human
history is marked by the
presence of beings who
help us to be more than we are.
We call these beings Angels.
We look for their
presence, but sometimes
forget to see.*

By the end of the first year when I was diagnosed with breast cancer, I continued to find myself in a place of rediscovery, and at times I felt like I was in limbo! I was a ship out at sea in the midst of a storm. I had a hard time going to work and I was still very fatigued. I kept asking my body to meet expectations that I knew it was unable to meet. I was not certain of where I was going and what I was going to do. At times, I felt that I was overly sensitive, especially at work, which may have caused more problems than really existed.

The things that I used to enjoy doing, I now had no energy to do, and it made me feel uneasy about myself. I wondered at times what was wrong with me, but I realized it was my fatigue and my priorities had changed. Living was taking on a new meaning, and what was important before seemed insignificant now. What is important is living a life that is full, and spending time with my spouse and children. As I have told those whom I work with, I want and need to make "good and happy memories."

I looked at our backyard and all the work we had put into it. I just don't want to take care of it anymore. I used to spend all my time outside planting, weeding, and watering, because it was a way for me to relieve tension and stress. It gave me pleasure and satisfaction. I would sit outside and admire what we had accomplished and the beauty of it all. I remember listening to the birds, and watching the butterflies and hummingbirds. While sitting on the patio, I would listen to my favorite music or relax in the pool, while I waited my husband to come home from work. It will always remain as work, but I will still enjoy the beauty.

I continued to look for that person who I was in the mirror's reflection. I saw imperfections and I just wished that I had my own breasts, or that these were so perfect that they looked like my own. One is larger than the other, but I am grateful that it is not recognizable when I am clothed. I can see and feel the implant in the reconstructed breast and I want to have it replaced. My husband says that I look just fine. I realize also, that some of my insecurity comes from the fact that he does not touch the reconstructed breast. He is afraid that he will hurt me. I know that if I had the implant replaced, that he may not even then, touch that breast.

I wonder sometimes if I want to have it replaced just because of vanity. I suppose that it could be considered vanity, and it probably is. I think that I just want things to be the way they were before, and I want my husband to feel comfortable and not fearful that he is going to hurt me. I had to realize that nothing would ever be the way that it was. It will never be the same. I would learn I was going to start a new life, and moments of tenderness would be my replacement for physical intimacy.

Being unable to accept my new body image is magnified because I never was proud of my appearance. I was teased in grade school and high school, so I was hesitant in being seen in a bathing suit, or without clothing. My present husband has never made me feel embarrassed or uncomfortable. I am trying to find a way to resolve this insecurity, because if I think that I look repulsive, then he must, too.

The person I was before the cancer arrived is still there. I have just been afraid to let her come out into the world. I think that I am trying to hide her for fear that she would be hurt again. I know that in order to love, we have to open ourselves up to the possibility of being hurt, and to have experiences that we might never have, just to learn from them. I learned that we are spirits from conception, brought into this world and given life within our present bodies. We are brought into this world to learn from our experiences. Lessons will repeat themselves until we learn what we are meant to learn. Learning why I had to develop breast cancer, and in the first fifteen months of my marriage was the lesson that I was to learn from.

As the weeks pass into months, I have found that I have strength that I did not know that I had. I see beauty in things that I never thought about before. I have learned how to connect my mind and body, and I feel an unusual sense of energy and peace within myself. The person I see in the mirror now, I know, is the same person, but with a desire to enjoy every moment, and to make memories and enjoy my family. Every moment, every day is a gift! I have learned to enjoy the extraordinary in the ordinary. I feel small when compared to the vastness of the Universe.

Losing my hair was also something I had to grieve. My hair was part of who I am, and losing it was devastating. When it started growing back, it grew in differently than I was accustomed to it looking. Then I just wanted it to grow really fast. When I went out in public, I often wondered if people were saying, "I bet she had cancer and chemotherapy." I felt that I had a sign on my forehead that flashed, "I had breast cancer."

I remembered what I looked like before, and now I had to make adjustments to this new look. I had to learn to accept it, but it was difficult. People told me that my hair was sassy, but I just wished that it would grow faster. I was fifty-two years young, and I did not want to have sassy hair. Every month I would ask my husband to take a picture of me so that I could see and have memories of the progressive hair growth. It is fun looking at old photographs to remember how I felt about the excitement or the sadness that I had had at the time. It allowed me to grow and become free, in a sense, from the devastating results of chemotherapy. It allowed me to know that I was and am a survivor.

I remember the first time I was able to feel the wind blow through my hair. There was a rush of excitement that filled my soul. I was sure that when people saw me standing with my arms in the air, turning around in a circle, smiling, and laughing, that they wondered if I had lost my mind. I will never have my hair cut again. When I had such a difficult time with losing my hair, my dear husband showed his softer side and said that he would shave his head so that it would look like mine. I was surprised by his sensitivity. I remember thanking him for offering his support, but I didn't want him to do it. I love his hair. It is white and light brown. His beard is white and he looks so distinguished. I don't know how many husbands offer to shave their heads, or even just do it so that they can be bald together. I was deeply touched with his offer of compassion and kindness. I knew how much he was hurting and how much he loved me.

My belly button did not heal the way that I had expected. I have a dimple. I was a little disappointed, but I realized that it was only a belly button. It was not as if I was twenty years old, wearing pants below the belly line, showing my mid-drift, or wearing a bikini. Dr. Geoffrey told me that he could revise the belly button, but since I had been poked, prodded, sliced and diced so many times, I just didn't want to have that procedure done.

I still have another surgery to go through. The doctors have deemed it a medical necessity that my ovaries be removed. Hopefully, that will end my need for surgeries, unless, of course, I decide that I want my breast revised . My husband does not want me to have another surgery. . Sometimes I feel like I am fluttering, like the leaves of a tree in the breeze. It is vanity that wants me to have it done so I can look as normal as possible. I wonder if not being able to see or feel the implant would make a difference in how I feel about myself.

As this last surgery approaches, I find myself becoming more anxious. I am worried that the incision will not heal. The surgeon would make the incision in the scar I already have, but that did not heal well. I went to see Dr. Geoffrey for a follow-up visit. As he sat in front of me, he looked at my breasts, and said that the scars were fading. He told me that after the surgery, I would be ready to have the tattooing done. I must have looked like I was having a bad day, because he asked what was going on with me. I told him that I was getting anxious about the upcoming surgery. I told him that I was worried that I might have the same problems with healing again, and I had a fear that they might find more cancer. He said that those thoughts were normal, but we also had to have positive thoughts, too. This surgery would prevent any chances of ovarian cancer. He said that it was very good that I had decided to go ahead with this, due to my mother's history of ovarian cancer.

I also told him about some burning and pulling-type pain that I had in my groin and that I thought it might be an inguinal hernia. He checked the area and he thought it might be a nerve trying to regenerate. He said that he could do a nerve block, but I wanted to wait to see if it would resolve on its own.

He remembered that I had the genetic testing done. He said he was glad that he had been in the office when I called. I was so upset because they told me that I would have to make a decision if I wanted to have a left breast mastectomy, a mammogram, and an ultrasound of the right breast every six months.

I think he was upset because he felt that the testing should have been done before the surgery, since it would have changed the initial course of treatment. He told me that I should just wait and see what the results showed. If I decided to have the mastectomy, he and his father would take care of it. I told him that no matter what the results of the testing showed, I had decided to take my chances and not have another mastectomy.

Even though the surgery was preventive, having another mastectomy would mean that I would still go through the same loss that I had gone through the first time. The grief may not have been with the same intensity, but I would still grieve. I would continue to look in the mirror, trying to find the person who I was before. There would be no sensation in either breast and that would affect our intimacy even more. I have spent so much time grieving and I am now just getting through this process. I do not want to start all over again. I began to cry and told him that I felt inadequate and guilty sometimes. I told him I am very angry because I don't have any sex drive, and my body does not respond to my husband's touch. I was single for twenty-one years, and raised my sons by myself. Then I found someone who I wanted to spend the rest of my life with, and now all this has happened. We were still in our honeymoon period, yet we were dealing with breast cancer and a mastectomy.

He took my hands and told me that I had been through a lot, and that I should not rush the decision. The desire and the ability to respond would come back. He said that it was probably too soon. Chemotherapy causes a lack of, or a decrease in the sex drive and ability to respond. He also reminded me that it had not even been a year since I had completed the treatment. He said that he understood it was difficult for me, but that I should not be so hard on myself. He suggested that I talk to my primary doctor because some women use Viagra. I told him that I had, and she had given me a prescription for a cream, but it wasn't very helpful.

He has not seen me too much in a state of mind that would show that I was healing emotionally. I think that is because I did not see him every day nor talk to him every day. Diana, my dear friend, a social worker, told me once that she could see that I was doing better because we talked every day. She said that I was making progress and appeared happier. I was beginning to laugh again and starting to enjoy life. I wanted him to see that I was doing better. I told him that I had written a book, and that it was going into production soon. I also told him that I had developed a web site. He was very excited, smiled, and gave me a hug. I told him that if the book only helped one person, then I had achieved my goal. He told me that it already had, because it had helped me. He stood up, smiled, and said, "No pictures today." I told him that I needed a few pictures of the two of us. I wanted to put them in my book. His face lit up and he smiled. He said, "Of course." He told me to look at his web site. There was pictures of Bonnie and the rest of his staff. I was excited because I would be able to share the faces of those who had supported me.

Then he held me, and told me that I was all right. He reminded me that I have been through a lot this past year, and that I needed to remember that I have just started a new life. I just have to be patient and not set my expectations too high. I will find a new sense of 'normal.' Boy! Where have I heard that before? He reaffirmed that I was strong and a survivor. "Helping others is something to be proud of. You will help more people than you realize at the moment." Again, he held me tight, and said, "I'm proud of you."

Most importantly for me, my doctor told me that our patient-doctor relationship was not over. He assured me that whenever I needed to talk to him, that I should call. He said that he would always be there to help me work through this. I told him that I didn't think that I would have been able to get through all that I have had to deal with, without his support and compassion. I really don't think that I could have, and that is why God led me to him, for He knew that I was going to need a compassionate, kind, and caring doctor. I was treated as a patient with breast cancer, and not as a breast cancer patient! There is a difference. It is important that when you are selecting your health care team, that they treat you as a patient, and not a diagnosis.

This was the first physician who ever took the time to talk to me about sexual relations with my husband, and I cherished his support and advice. My primary physician has talked to me about this, but the oncologist actually did not want to hear anything about it. He suggested that I see my gynecologist.

I thought about how much I cared for Dr. Geoffrey, for my husband, and for my friends who have stood by me. The word 'care' haunted me so much that I had to look up its meaning. Care has its roots in the Gothic *Kara,* meaning to grieve, experience sorrow, and to cry out. I realized if a person truly cares, they must join with the person in pain, whether that's through the emotional or physical realms. Sometimes that is all that can be done. My family, husband, friends, and Dr Geoffrey shared my pain, my sorrow. They encouraged me to allow myself to grieve, and reminded me that I should not hurry - the process of healing. Henri Nouwen, in his book, *Out of Solitude,* says, ". . . when we honestly ask ourselves which person in our lives means the most to us, we often find it is those who, instead of giving advice, solutions or cures, have chosen rather to share our pain, and touch our wounds with a gentle and tender hand."

The friends who can be silent with us in a moment of despair or confusion, who can stay with us in an hour of grief or bereavement, who can tolerate not knowing, not curing, and not healing, while still facing us with the reality of our powerlessness, those are the friends who care. They are the ones who want to share our journey with us. Sharing our journey with those who want to listen, is how we heal.

With that thought in mind, I believe it is for that reason that my family, friends, and Dr. Geoffrey mean so much to me and have been able to help me through this journey. As a support team, they have listened without placing judgment, and without giving advice. Dr. Geoffrey let his human side be his guide, and supported me through some of the roughest times that I have had to endure. Diana, LouAnne, and Dr. Geoffrey shared their unique selves with me, which in essence, is where I gathered my strength to be a survivor.

I got home and my husband, Wayne, was sitting in the chair. I told him about my visit with Dr. Geoffrey. I started to cry and he held me. I just sobbed uncontrollably. I told him that I feel so helpless and alone sometimes. I told him that I wished that we could go back to where we were before all this started. He said that we would get back there. He told me that he was not disappointed in me, and I was everything that he ever wanted.

Later in the month, he told me that I was dwelling too much on this "sex thing" as he called it. I needed to let it go. He compared this to his recent shoulder operation, and said that he was not going to let the pain or fear control him. I was angry! I just lost a body part—a body part that society looks at as part of a woman's sexual attractiveness. It had been a physical part of me, and part of our past sexual experiences. I have had to face a life threatening disease that caused my body image to change. We were losing interest in our sexual life and he wanted me to let it go? Did he truly believe I could stop dwelling on it? How could I possibly do that? I was confused. Didn't our sex life mean anything to him? Was that particular part of our relationship meaningless? He just didn't understand because he had not been threatened with any disease that could eventually lead to death.

I could not talk with him about this for awhile. I was too upset and angry. I had to wait, collect my thoughts, and not get too emotional about what he had said. As I thought about it, I realized he wanted me to feel less pressure about it. He had just used the wrong choice of words to relieve any anxiety that I had. As I thought about what he had said, I knew that he was right. I needed to "let go." I could rely on his strength, and believe that I meant just as much to him now as before, and probably more. Having lost a breast had not really changed anything at all. I had to rebuild my confidence and self-esteem.

I finally sat down and talked to him. I told him how I felt about the statement that he had made when he said I was dwelling too much on this "sex thing." He was hurt that I would even think that he thought our sexual relationship was meaningless. As expected, he was hoping to make me feel less pressured. He said that it would all come back in time and we would find ourselves where we were before.

I miss the closeness that we had had before all this started a year ago. Resolving sexual problems is difficult in any marriage. Now we were not only dealing with that, but it has been caused by a life-threatening disease. We were still newlyweds, and we were dealing with breast cancer, our emotions and feelings, the changes in my appearance, and trying to find a way to re-learn how to enjoy our sex life. It is a burden that both partners must share. The reality of my sex drive never returning, frightened me, but I realized that it may take longer to arouse me. There is comfort in knowing that I have the desire to be with my husband, and there is comfort in knowing that he wants to be with me. It is just a matter of re-learning and being comfortable.

I keep a diary of when I think about sex. I want to know what I am feeling at the time, what I was imagining or fantasizing about, and if anything happened. Did we have intimacy? I searched for specific times or days that the thought crossed my mind, so that I would have some idea when it would be good for me to attempt having relations with my husband. For awhile, there were no thoughts about it at all. Then, I noticed when reviewing the entries in my diary, that at some moments the idea of having sex was there, but nothing happened.

It has been a year, and I have noticed that my thoughts of sex are more frequent. When I go to bed at night, I do think about being kissed, touched, and caressed. I am beginning to feel excitement, thinking about being with my husband, but I am still reluctant to try. I don't want either of us to be disappointed or become frustrated.

I have not discussed this with him yet. I have thought maybe the next step would be to just lie in each other's arms, touch each other, and actually find places on our bodies that stimulate one another. Massage is very stimulating and it would also be relaxing. It sounds very self-centered. I am not sure that my husband would understand that because he would not want to be self-centered with me.

I know in my heart that I need to know if I can still excite him with my touch and that he will become excited when he touches me. Using oils, lighting aromatic candles, and setting a romantic atmosphere may help. Our tastes in music are very different but playing soft romantic music would also help set the mood. There is never a good time for intimacy, so we will have to make the time. When we are both home and if the desire comes, we will have to make the time right at that moment. We will not be able to say not now, or later. It will have to be then because the desire may not be there later.

Most men do not know how to talk to women when it comes to sensitive things like sex. They think we should be able to read their minds. We, on the other hand, want to hear words that will support and validate how we feel. We want to know that they understand. I think as women, we speak with our heads and hearts, and men just speak with their heads. They try to be strong and don't realize at that moment that we need them to open their hearts and be sensitive and "touchy-feely" with us. They probably think that we need to grow up! I think about this as I am writing and I start to laugh. This is so typical and normal. Women want to be talked to with emotions, and men just assume that their spouses know how they feel. I have a dear friend who told me that she tells her husband that when he is being sensitive, or "touchy-feely" with her, that it is "foreplay, baby!" I think that is just so wonderful!

Soon I would discover that he had fears other than losing me. He was afraid to have sex and afraid to touch me. He thought that he would hurt me. In a few months, he would be able to talk to me about his fears of being intimate. As we discuss how we feel, and spend time together, we find that we must learn how to make love to each other again. We have to guide each other's hands, without words, and teach each other what feels good. We could not be shy, or hesitant, inhibited. If we wanted to work at saving our marriage we would have to teach each other what we liked and disliked.

Later in the year, we were going to bed separately. Months would pass without touching, kissing or holding each other. If there was a moment of intimacy, I discovered that I had lost all sensation everywhere, including in my left breast and pelvic area.

He works later all the time. Then he comes home, eats dinner and falls asleep in the chair. When he says that he is planning to go into the pool, I get ready and wait for him. He never joins me. Later, when I am busy doing something else, he says he is going out to the pool. I just feel that he is happier when he is not around me. I worry about where our relationship is headed and if we need to see a counselor.

I realized I was responsible for my guilt and inadequate feelings. I needed to give myself more time. I needed to be patient and give him more time to work through his fears, his grieving. It wasn't only due to the physical effects of surgery and treatment. It was me not accepting my new body image and fearing that I was no longer physically attractive to my husband. It was the result of a long history of not being proud of how I looked when I was younger. Time is the essence of healing. I had to stop setting expectations that pressured me. I needed to go back to taking one day at a time.

With the next surgery only four days away, I acknowledged that I had allowed a cloud to hang over my head. That corner reserved in my mind for "cancer worry" which ebbs like the tide, had filled my life. I felt like I was smothering in fear. Crying had become very easy. I sat down and started to write about why I was afraid.

There were many things that came to mind, but I realized that with everything that I had gone through during the past year, it was all right to be scared. I just needed to stop, and remove the big "E" (expectations) off my forehead. I could not expect to erase all that happened in the past year. I could not expect to go back to work two weeks after surgery. It is normal to fear that the biopsy report will show cancer. Ovarian cancer is the silent killer. It is diagnosed when it is too late. My husband wanted me to cancel the surgery because I was scared. I explained that I couldn't do that and I told him why. With my mother's history and now with the breast cancer, I did not want to take that chance.

I have not been this scared since all this started a year ago. I was not scared about the mastectomy until it was all done. Afterwards, in the hospital, was when the fear began to set in. Lying in the darkness in my hospital bed I realized what had just taken place and what the future was going to hold for my family and myself.

I drove to the hospital for the pre-operative paperwork and blood tests. My heart was pounding and my chest felt empty. Tears started running down my cheeks. I filled out the history forms and had to write down the surgeries I have had over the years. It took me several minutes before I could write breast cancer, right mastectomy in May, 2004. I wanted to cry. When the nurse began asking me questions, I realized that I had not remembered to write down some things. I was embarrassed, but I realized that it was "brain fog" from the fibromyalgia, and maybe some short-term memory loss from the chemotherapy. More fear began to set in. Was I losing my mind as well, or it the result of all the surgeries and the chemotherapy? Was it just from stress?

As I drove to work after I had completed everything, I started crying again. I told myself I was scared and I recited the reasons why. While at work, I decided to write about my feelings. As I wrote, I discovered the only true fear I had was wondering if the biopsy would be positive. If it was, what would I do? How would my husband and sons react? I did not know the answers to those questions, and

I realized that I could not feel for them. I had no control over the outcome. I had to stay positive and acknowledge that those fears were normal. I was reminded that each time a symptom appeared or whenever I got sick, that the "cancer worry" would return to the forefront of my mind.

We always hear and are told that, "God does not give us more than we can handle." I have been tested beyond my ability to cope at times. I tell anyone who recites that verse to me that they have no idea what it is like. They have not endured what I, and many others have had to endure with this devastating disease! They do not know how they will react if it happens to them. I originally thought I was okay with it. It was just a breast! But I wasn't okay with it. Now I continue the fight to survive and deal with other situations that come along at the same time.

I talked to Judy, a friend whom I work with, and we decided that she would hypnotize me. We went to the quiet room and I closed my eyes. I breathed deeply and concentrated on her voice. All the other sounds became distant, and all I heard was her voice, soft and steady. She took me to a place in my mind where I felt comfortable. There was a stream with the sound of water running over rocks. I sat under a tree with the sun on my face, and colorful flowers all around me. I became one with the chair that I was sitting in.

She surrounded me with colors and I saw a figure come to me. It was Wayne, my husband. She wanted to know what he was saying. I told her that he said that he would always be with me. She told me that I was worthy and safe, that he was my true soul mate, and that I would heal and have peace. She was able to take me to other places of comfort and peace.

She brought me back and told me that my trigger word was "peach bubble" and when I felt myself getting anxious and worried, that I should say the trigger word. It would take me to that place where I found comfort and peace. This was one of the most exciting experiences of the mind-spirit life that I have ever known! When I feel myself getting nervous, or feeling unworthy and confused, I say those words. It immediately puts me in a trance where I am surrounded by this peach bubble and I feel safe.

When Wayne got home from work that night, I told him about this experience. I was so excited and he said that he was glad that it worked for me. We had talked about having Judy hypnotize him for weight control. I asked him if he thought he would be able to empty his mind of any thoughts. Could he concentrate on her voice and let the sounds outside fade away? He said he didn't think so. He is an electrical engineer, and they are always thinking. I am not sure how he even sleeps because he is always thinking.

I continue to have discomfort in my abdomen from the mastectomy and reconstruction of the breast. Dr. Geoffrey told me that it would last about nine months, and here it is nearly a year later and I still hurt. Sometimes I think maybe the cancer has come back or maybe it was there all along and nobody knew. There were no ultrasounds or gastrointestinal studies done, because I had no symptoms to even suggest that there was a problem. It sounds like I have become a hypochondriac, but I believe that I have become more aware of what is going on in my body. The "cancer worry" is still there.

I went to the Virginia Piper Cancer Center for the genetic testing that my oncologist wanted me to have completed. They explained to me that I would have to document my family tree, to the best of my abilities, complete with the causes of death, and at what age. I would also have blood work done that would allow them to test the genes to search for defects. With a defect present, it would place me in the thirty-to-forty percentile for the reoccurrence of the breast cancer, or to develop lung, bone or liver cancer. I wasn't sure that I wanted to know, because it would place added stress and worry on my family and myself. Knowing the results would not change anything that may happen in the future. I would not be able to change the course of my longevity.

When I saw and spoke with the oncologist, I felt some relief. I don't have to see him for another three to four months. We discussed having scans but he said that he doesn't like to do nuclear scans unless there are symptoms. He felt that introducing radioactive material was more harmful than not doing them. He ordered blood work and a bone density scan. He was waiting on the results of the genetic testing.

My calcium was a little low and he wanted to know what the bone density results were before he changed any medications. I was already taking calcium and he told me not to lift weights or do strenuous exercise, and to be careful walking. The Arimidex causes osteoporosis and I could have spontaneous fractures.

I told him that I was just diagnosed with fibromyalgia and that I needed to walk and was having massage and Jacuzzi therapy every week. He said that was really good and should be helpful. He asked if the Motrin was helping the muscle pain, and I told him that it was. I felt good about this oncologist. He took the time to talk to me and answered my questions. He always tells me that if I have any problems or questions to call him. It gives me comfort to know that I have someone who is watching over me, caring about what I am thinking and how I am feeling. He doesn't make me feel he is rushed or that he doesn't have time.

Sometimes I wonder when it will all end. Will I ever feel healthy and good again? Sometimes I do not see any end in sight. I am forever hurting, and cannot sleep through the night because of the pain in my muscles. I bought a couple of books on fibromyalgia so I can learn about the disease. I want to learn how to feel better again, and learn how to deal with the disease and the pain. The worst part of having fibromyalgia is that no one believes you. No one knows the pain that is involved.

With surgery soon approaching, I am worried that I will have to be off work longer than two weeks. I need to return to work because any longer than two weeks will result in a greater financial strain. We would have to pay Cobra to keep our health insurance, and because it is such an excellent policy, the monthly cost is nearly $1,000.00. I called the gynecologist and explained why I needed to go back to work early. He said that as long as there were no complications, that he would write a letter to release me. I then called Dr. Geoffrey to be sure that he would agree to release me in two weeks. He said that it would be all right with him.

The spouse is often a forgotten participant in this journey. Wayne has never spoken about how he feels since we were forced to take this journey so early in our marriage. One Sunday, just as we were finishing dinner, we started talking about the upcoming surgery. He said that he had lost faith in the doctors. He thought they were using these surgeries as a means to make more money. I got upset and said, "I made the choice to have surgery. I did not have to go through all this."

He said, "You did need to have the surgery, but we were told that the cancer was localized to the nipple. They said you would not need chemotherapy, and then the oncologist said that you did. Now they are saying that you need to have your ovaries removed."

I was sitting in the chair and he apologized. He said that it was all the stress and he just became angry. I told him it was all right to be angry. I started to cry because today I felt very unworthy and unattractive. I tried to have intimacy with him today and I felt like a failure. I could not physically respond to his touch. I feel pleasure in meeting his physical needs. I cannot help feeling that I am not meeting his needs because I cannot become stimulated, or excited by his touch. I asked him if this was part of what he was angry about. He denied it, and said that I should not feel like a failure.

"It will come back," he said, "and if it doesn't, we will deal with it."

I think that it is not only the loss of sensation, but as I have stated before, I am not comfortable with the way that I look. If both breasts were the same size, and if the tattooing was complete, maybe I would be more comfortable. I am also in constant pain and I know that makes it impossible for me to relax. Maybe it is just pride and vanity that will not allow me to accept the appearance of my breasts as they are. Even if it is, I need to be happy with the way I look. What I do need to remember though, is that I am still a woman. I am still full of life, having wants and desires. If I am going to have the revision done because of vanity or pride, it is ALL RIGHT!

Thinking about my appearance, I thought about my high school days and early adulthood. At that time, we were concerned with our appearance, sex appeal, and having a body that was desirable. I was always on the heavy side and self-conscious of how I looked. Our society and peers put that pressure on us.

I thought I had outgrown that type of thinking, but by losing a breast, I had to face my own mortality. My rationalization is that because I look different, I have gone back to that early adulthood thinking. Maybe because I am a newlywed, my physical appearance means more to me. My husband, however, does not think that I look any different. He would rather have me alive and with him. He does not care whether I have one or two breasts. He tells me all the time that he thinks I am beautiful. He has never done or said anything that would suggest he thought any other way. It has been me who has had the problem.

The day before the surgery, I got a letter from my dad and stepmother. My dad had been diagnosed with bone cancer. I had not seen or spoken to him in nearly thirty years. I do not understand what happened when my parents got divorced, but it seemed that my dad wanted to separate himself from me and my sister.

I thought about not having a father throughout all these past years, and I wondered how he must by not having developed a relationship with his daughters, or his grandchildren. There were so many things that we had all missed. I was not angry, and I don't ever remember being angry. I was just sad. It may have been helpful to me if we would not have been estranged all these years. Perhaps he could have supported me during this past year. I often wondered after I wrote and told him about the breast cancer diagnosis, what he felt. Did he regret not having a loving relationship, would he have been there to support me?

I told my husband that I had to go home and see him. I had to do this for dad and for myself. Whatever was said or not said in the past, did not matter anymore. What mattered was that we had to resolve the situation and forgive one another, so that we could pass from this life to another, knowing that we loved each other. We should not have to depart from this world with the guilt of "only if" I had done something before he died. I had to mend the gap that had come between us.

We made plans to go back to Toledo and spend some time with my son and his girlfriend. I wrote to my dad and told him when we would be there. I told him we would like to come see him. I sent him a copy of the book I had written, and told him that I thought he would like to read it. He was a very private person, unemotional, and had never talked with my sister or me much when we lived at home. Even though I wanted to see him, I was nervous about it. I was not sure what I was going to say, or what he would say. I was sure that he would not bring up what had happened so many years ago. He had written before that sometimes it is best to leave some things unsaid.

On Tuesday, at 5:00 a.m., we drove to the hospital. Wayne was nervous. His voice and hands were shaking as we waited in the registration lobby for them to call my name. I signed some papers and then we walked to the holding lobby until they were ready for me. We were taken into another holding area and they took my height, weight, and vital signs. Then I was given a paper gown and slippers to put on.

Now I was the one getting nervous. I had my worry stone with me and I was rubbing it continuously. It was cold in the holding area and they gave me a couple of warmed blankets. The nurse asked more questions and then started me on an IV. She poked and prodded at my hand until I thought I was going to scream. The hand she had to use was used for chemotherapy and the veins were collapsed and very difficult to find. I asked her to start it in my left arm, but she would not listen. I was getting angry!

Diana finally arrived and we hugged one another. The three of us sat and talked until the surgeon came. She is a good person. She is overwhelmed with a heavy caseload but she never lets her patients or families know. She will stop what she is doing and go see them if they are having a difficult time. Now here she was, very busy with patients and families, and she was sitting with us! She talked to us and supported us. There appeared to be nothing else on her mind but to give us the emotional support that we needed. Secretly, Diana knew my fear was that they would find cancer. I never told Wayne that I had been thinking about it, but it weighed heavy on his mind, too. He did not want me to go through another surgery. He did not want me to be in pain.

Diana was always available when I needed her. I could talk to her, and she understood what I felt. She had a similar experience and she helped me understand why I felt the way that I did and she helped me work through my fears. Diana came to the office at least twice a week, not only to drop off her paperwork, but to spend time with me. She is a true friend. She listens and sometimes does not say a word, but just holds me. That is true friendship. She is willing to walk this journey with me without placing judgment, with silence and she doesn't give advice. She gives encouragement and validates my feelings.

The nurse from the operating room came to ask me some questions. I knew that the time was fast approaching. Dr. Brachfeld arrived, and he was smiling. He is tall, probably about six-foot-five, has dark hair and a nice firm handshake. I introduced him to Wayne. I asked if I could go home after surgery and he said that I would be in the hospital for two days. I smiled and said that I was only trying. I remembered that when I first went to see him and was in the waiting room, that he came out to get me himself. I knew then that he was passionate about what he did and had compassion for his patients.

I was getting even more nervous because Dr. Geoffrey was not there yet. The anesthesiologist came and I was able to joke around with him. He asked if I was getting anxious and I started to laugh. I told him to bring on the "happy drugs." He laughed. He asked some questions and then wanted to know when was the last time that I had something to eat or drink. I told him it had been 8:00 p.m. on the previous day and it wasn't fair that he was standing there with my favorite coffee (Starbucks) and I couldn't have any.

He laughed and said to me, "You really need some happy drugs don't you? I am going to get you something to help you relax." He came back with the medication and the nurse was there. Dr. Geoffrey still had not come. I was sitting up on the gurney and tears started to run down my face. I wanted to see him before they took me into the surgical suite. Just as I said that, Dr. Geoffrey came around the corner, smiling. I felt such a sense of relief. He shook hands with Wayne and then gave me a hug. He asked if I had gotten his message last week. I told him that I had, and I thanked him. He started to pull the curtain. Wayne got up to leave and Dr. Geoffrey told him he didn't need to leave. Wayne said he knew that, but he wanted to leave.

He was looking for something and then I realized that he was looking for a marker. I love this man, in spite of his markers and camera! The funny thing is though, I expect it each time I see him. He drew on my belly where he was going to revise the scar, and then he touched what was to have been my belly button. He said we would talk about this later. Tears ran down my face. I sat up and he held me. He said that I would be all right. I told him that I was so glad that he was going to be there with me. It gave me comfort that he probably didn't understand. To my surprise, he said that he did understand. We had been through a lot together. His compassion just filled me with peace!

They started taking me to the surgical suite and they almost didn't let me kiss my husband. I started to panic because I couldn't find him, and then there he was! He towered over me, and told me that he loved me and would see me later. Crying, I put my arms around his neck, and told him I loved him with all my heart and soul.

The surgical suite was white, barren, and cold. All the huge equipment was overwhelming and frightening. I was amused at myself because I remembered that I was a nurse and this is a normal surgical suite. I also knew that I was once again on the other side of the medical chart. I wasn't a nurse. I was a patient. They had me move over to the surgery table. I asked for a warm blanket, but didn't get one. The nurses were not friendly. They were busy getting everything ready for the surgeons. They took my left arm out of the gown and put a blood pressure cuff on. Then I was told that an oxygen mask was being placed on my face. I asked for Dr. Geoffrey. I remember saying, "Where is Dr Geoffrey?" Then he came up to me on my right side and took my hand. He was holding it tight. Tears ran down my face. I was scared of the unknown. I heard him tell the anesthesiologist to wait. He bent down and wiped the tears from my face and told me that I was going to be all right.

I don't remember being taken to my room, and I don't recall either Dr. Brachfeld or Dr. Geoffrey coming to see me in recovery. I remember Wayne putting my wedding rings on and sitting down beside me. I asked if everything was okay and he told me that Dr. Brachfeld said that he had had a hard time. He couldn't find the left ovary and almost stopped the surgery. However, he decided to look some more. He found it under the bowel lying up against the pancreas. He said that they looked normal. He told me that there were a lot of adhesions and I would be pretty uncomfortable because he had to move things around in there.

I remember telling Wayne to go home and get something to eat, to take care of the dogs and come back later. I went to sleep. When I woke up, I wanted to thank

Dr. Geoffrey. I called Sheila at his office and asked her to tell him thank you. She said that he was there and he picked up the phone. He said that he had come into recovery but I was too sleepy. He said that it was good that he was there, because Dr. Brachfeld had a hard time. He repeated what Wayne had told me and then said that everything looked good. If his schedule permitted, he said he would stop by to see me the next day. Otherwise, I was to see him the following Tuesday. I told him thank you and he said that it was his pleasure to help.

Wayne came back that evening and I had already been up walking. Then we went for a walk. I think that I even walked several times more that night. At 4:00 a.m., they removed the foley catheter and by 6:00 a.m., I was up going to the bathroom and had cleaned up by myself. I took another walk. Dr. Brachfeld came in. I told him that I had been walking and they removed the foley catheter, and that I was going to the bathroom. He said that I could go home tomorrow. I was disappointed, so I asked if I could go home today? He asked if I was passing gas. I told him I was and he said, "Home you go!" He sat on the bed and looked at the incision that Dr. Geoffrey had made. He asked what said the doctor had told me, and I said all I knew was that I was to see him next Tuesday.

I thanked him for taking care of me, and we began to talk about physicians having passion, about what they do, and compassion for their patients. I told him the story about finding Dr. Robert and Dr. Geoffrey Leber. I told him I felt that Dr. Robert had sent me to him because he had passion for his work and compassion for his patients. He smiled and said thank you. He said that he did have passion for what he does. I told him that God had guided me to the best surgeons that I could possibly have, and for that I thanked Him every day!

It has now been nearly a week since surgery, and I am going to see the genetic counselor for the results of the testing. Surprisingly, I am not worried. I am not sure why. Before, I was afraid that the testing would be positive, and now that I know my father has bone cancer, I am sure that it will be positive. I did some research and found that the majority of people do come back positive, whether it's genetic or environmental. I think that maybe I am calm about it because it is not going to change what I have decided to do for follow-up. Whatever plans God has for me, I will trust that He will help me through it.

As I drove to the Virginia Piper Center for Cancer Research, I just enjoyed the ride. I listened to old love songs and some jazz. I didn't have any trouble parking. As I walked into the lobby, and let them know that I was there for my appointment, I saw several women wearing caps and hats. They had lost their hair from chemotherapy. It brought back the feelings that I had. I felt myself withdrawing and beginning to worry about the test results. I closed my eyes and breathed deeply to relax, and thought of my safe place that Judy had given me when I was getting worried.

The counselor came into the lobby and took me to a conference room. I explained that Wayne could not be there because they had an emergency power problem and he was not able to leave. I sat down and she explained the testing once again. Then she gave me a piece of paper. As I read it, she said that the testing did not show any mutation of the genes. I did not receive the chromosome from my mother, even though she had cancer at a very young age.

I was speechless. I could not believe what I was hearing. I was sure that it was going to show there were mutated genes, and that I would be at high risk of developing cancer somewhere else in my body! The oncologist came in, introduced herself and said that the testing was good. They did not know what caused breast cancer. She said that having my ovaries removed and taking the Arimidex, with close follow-up with my oncologist, was proving beneficial. She did advice me to have a colonoscopy done every year. (That procedure was already scheduled at the request of my primary care physician.)

When I left, I remained somewhat in a state of disbelief. I decided to drive to my husband's plant and tell him my news in person. As I drove, I began to think and wonder about the color therapy and meditation that Jan and Judy had me do whenever I was worried. I wondered if breathing in green mist and watching it encircle around my body, feeling its energy as it left my fingers, really worked. Or, was it just that it was detected early, and the chemotherapy worked? Was it an unknown factor that caused the breast cancer? Could it have been the stress that we had been under that first year and the estrogen replacement therapy?

I waited for Wayne to come to the lobby. He came in through the front door because he had been outside and had seen my truck. He asked what was wrong. I went outside with him and told him about the test results. He kept repeating, no mutations! No mutations! There was relief and excitement in his voice, and it showed on his face. I started to cry and he held me tight. His hands were shaking, he was so happy.

I cannot describe the feeling that I had when I heard that the tests proved normal. I think because of the results, I will be able to complete my emotional recovery at a steady pace. I will have more good days than bad days. I will laugh more often, but I know that I will continue to laugh through my tears. I will be able to obtain that inner peace that I have been searching for.

With all the research and medical technology, still, no one knows what causes breast cancer. There appears to be a relationship between hormone replacement, stress, and the development of breast cancer. Some doctors are trying to take their patients off hormone replacement therapy. Having had all the symptoms of menopause, I had a very difficult time, until I started hormone replacement. Now, given the choice, I think that I would try natural remedies instead, after having gone through all that I have. However, that may not have prevented developing breast cancer. We went out to dinner that night and all Wayne could say was "that news was worth a million dollars!" He could not be any happier than he was right then. I knew just how deeply this had touched him, and just how frightened he was.

It was a Tuesday morning when I had my follow-up appointment with Dr. Brachfeld. I needed to be released to go to work the following Monday. The nurse took me to the examining room and gave me a cotton sheet. I was told to remove my clothing from the waist down because she didn't know if he would want to do a pelvic exam so soon after the surgery.

I was sitting on the exam table when Dr. Brachfeld knocked and came in. He smiled, said hi and asked how I was doing. I told him that I was doing good, had very little discomfort, but I was still tired. He asked what I was doing there so soon. I told him that I needed to go back to work on Monday. He helped me lie down on the table and gently did an abdominal exam, but he didn't do a pelvic exam. He wanted Dr. Geoffrey to remove the steri-strips from the incision. He said that I was amazing. I told him that I didn't know about that, and he said yes, you are! I could not understand why he said that I was amazing.

He helped me sit up and then he sat on a stool to look at the pathology report. He read it and then told me that the right ovary was normal. The left ovary, the only words that come to mind to make it easy to understand, were pre-cancerous. He said that it was a good thing that I had them removed. Tears started to well up in my eyes. My heart hit my feet, or at least that is how I felt.

I told him that I had a question about my inability to respond to my husband physically when we wanted to be intimate. He sat and looked at me tentatively. I told him that I knew that I would not have any sex drive, but I did want to be able to respond to my husband. He asked if I could be aroused by clitoris stimulation. I told him that it took a very long time. I thought that my husband was as frustrated as I was.

He smiled and said that there was nothing wrong with taking a long time making love. He told me to think about it, and it could really be a good thing. I also needed to remember that the older we get, the longer it does take to be aroused.

He then told me that he could not give me any testosterone because that converts to estrogen. I should not allow anyone to try and give it to me. He then asked if we had tried a vibrator. I told him no, and I wasn't sure that I could do that. He wanted to know why. I told him that it made me feel uncomfortable and embarrassed. He told me there was nothing to be embarrassed about and even young girls used them. He said it would help, and that we needed to take our time making love.

I lowered my head and tears started to run down my face. I told him that I just felt inadequate. He asked if we had had a good sexual relationship before the breast cancer. I told him that we did. His question then was, what about now? I explained that we seldom have intimacy. He replied that using a vibrator was even more important now, so that we could resume our intimacy. Sex is a very important part of a relationship and there was no reason that we could not have the same active sexual relationship that we did before. He continued to say that even though we are at an age where sexual activity usually declines, we are still newlyweds, and that it is important we stay active until there is a natural decline in our sexual relationship. He reassured me that I didn't need to feel inadequate. He repeated that I was a remarkable woman and that most women will not even talk to their GYN about their sex problems. He thanked me for doing so. He also gave me a card for a store that one of his patients runs that sells vibrators. He held me and said that I need not be embarrassed. He told me that I needed to remember that I am a remarkable woman and I had been through a lot. He reinforced that I needed to be patient and slow in making love.

I called to tell Wayne what he said, but he wasn't available. I left him a message and told him to call me. I really didn't want to tell him over the phone that the ovaries were removed just in time. I felt elated, but concerned, because I did not know exactly what that meant. I was letting my imagination take over and thought it would mean more chemotherapy. The nurse in me did not surface this time! I called Diana and asked her to call me. She returned my call right away and said that I didn't sound so good. I told her what the pathology report said and I started to cry. She asked what it meant, and I told her that I really didn't know. They were going to send the report to the oncologist. She told me to stay off the Internet! She knew that I would start researching before I saw the oncologist, and I would get myself in another state of fearfulness. She suggested that I should make an appointment with the oncologist as soon as possible to get some answers. She reminded me that my ovaries were gone, and it may not mean anything now. After we talked, the nurse in me came to the surface. I told myself that I was being silly because I knew that everything was all right. I was okay and would not need chemotherapy.

I talked to Wayne when he got home after dinner about all that Dr. Brachfeld had said. I had a difficult time discussing the use of a vibrator. To my surprise, he said he thought it was a good idea and that we would go together and get one. He told me something that impacted my thoughts. He said that he would rather I be alive and well without the ability of having sex, rather than living without me in his life.

I believe though, as a woman, we need to have that physical closeness. Otherwise, we just don't feel good about ourselves, and the relationship we are in. If there is a joint decline with age and we have been in a relationship for a long time, we understand better the other means of being close and sexual. As a newlywed, and then having a life-threatening disease and body changes, I was fearful that I was no longer sexually attractive. I needed to have that closeness even more. I found the courage to go to the store that Dr. Brachfeld suggested to buy a vibrator. I was very uncomfortable and embarrassed.

A young man came up to me and wanted to help me as I stood at the desk. But I told him that I wanted to speak to the girl behind the counter. She came over and I told her what had happened and why I was there. I also told her that I knew nothing about this kind of thing and I needed her assistance. She said that she understood and that I should not be embarrassed. She said that she understood that I was from a generation that did not use them, and if women at my age did not reach orgasm, then it was just the way it was. She said that this would help me and that eventually I may not even need to use it. We went to the vibrator section of the store, and she showed me two different kinds. I asked her which one was best. I didn't know what would be best for me.

The next question in my mind was how to use this "toy" as she called it, when I was in the process of making love, but I could not ask her that. I knew that Wayne and I would have to figure that one out for ourselves.

I told my husband that I bought the vibrator and showed it to him. He started to make jokes and was laughing hysterically. I got upset, and I started to cry, holding my head down. I told him that I was not happy about this, but I wanted to be able to enjoy sex again. I told him that I bought this thing for us, and that I didn't know how or when to use it. I said that I didn't think it was something to laugh about.

He apologized and said that he didn't know how or when to use it, either, but that we would figure it out together. He wanted to be able to have me enjoy sex, too, and not become so frustrated anymore. He said that he understood the importance that this had for me because of losing my breast, and that I didn't feel complete and he would help me.

I thought about his reaction and I understood that he was just as nervous about using this "toy" as I was. It was foreign to both of us and we would have to learn together, so neither of us would feel uncomfortable. It was all about what makes each of us comfortable and giving each other pleasure in our sexual life. When I was alone thinking about this, I started to laugh. Here we were at fifty-some years of age, and we didn't know how to use a vibrator. We must be living in the dark ages! Or, we just lived very sheltered lives!

I was hoping that we would be able to have some time together this weekend, but it didn't turn out that way. He fell asleep in the chair and I fell asleep on the bed. When it was nine in the evening, he went to bed and I was sitting at the computer writing. As I wrote, I wondered if we were just avoiding each other. I started to laugh at myself, because my husband had been working twelve hours a day, and six days a week. Who wouldn't be too tired?

Now I would have to tell my sons about the pathology report. I don't like falling apart when I talk to them. I have always been strong for them, but I guess that I need to accept the fact that they are adults. I can't hide them from the fear and the pain. They are now my "rock" as I have always been for them.

I spoke to all three of my sons. There was a big sigh of relief when I told them that it was not cancerous now but would have been soon. They asked if I was all right, and I told them that I was fine and going back to work on Monday. I told them I didn't want to, but I didn't have any choice because of the health insurance. I didn't tell them that there was a corner in my mind that was making me anxious, because I didn't know for certain that I would not need chemotherapy again, or if it just meant that it was over.

I went to see Dr. Geoffrey. He apologized and I asked him what for? He said that he was trying to come to see me on Wednesday but that he was so busy. I told him not to apologize since I went home that morning. He asked how I was doing and I told him I was doing good, and that Dr. Brachfeld left the steri-strips for him to remove. He told me that it was a difficult surgery and that they could not find the left ovary because it was so small and the right one was benign. I told him that Dr. Brachfeld told me that it had some cysts and that the pathology report said that it was precancerous. His face showed disbelief, and he said "someone up there wants you around for a while." (Three weeks after the surgery, I found out from one of our medical directors, that there was nothing to worry about.)

Dr. Salvatore is a radiology oncologist and he stopped in my office to see how I was doing. I had asked about the biopsy and what that meant for me. He smiled and said that it meant I was okay now. He told me to call him anytime I had questions, day or night. I thought how kind that was of him, and supportive. I now have another person in my support system. I e-mailed Wayne at work and told him what Dr. Salvatore said and he was as relieved as I was. I didn't have to wait until my next oncology appointment to find out if I was all right or if I was going to need more chemotherapy.

I had to go back to see Dr. Geoffrey, and he examined the suture line. He said that it was a little uneven but it was still under the bikini line. I told him that I wasn't going to be wearing any bikini. He smiled and said, "You never know!" He left the steri-strips on and said that he wanted to see me in three weeks. If they were still on, he would remove them.

He looked at the reconstructed breast where the tissue is very thin, and he was not happy. He said that he was concerned about it. If it opened, I would need to come to his office right away and he could close it. If I could see the implant at any time, that meant he would have to remove it , allow it to heal, and then he would do the revision.

He looked at what should have been a belly button and apologized that it didn't work out as planned. He said that when I was ready, he had a couple of ideas that would work to make it better. If I wanted him to do that, then he would revise the breast, and redo the belly button at the same time. It would be out-patient surgery so I would not have to stay overnight .

He asked if I was ready to have the tattooing done and I told him that I was. He said he would have Bonnie send me the information. He thought trying to match it with the other side would be the best way, but if it didn't work then they would make it a darker color on both sides so that they did match. He gave me a hug and told me to call him if I needed anything at all. I smiled and thanked him for being such a kind and compassionate person. He told me that he wanted me to be happy with the way I looked and knew that it was important to me.

After a week, I had decided that in June, I would have him revise the breast. I know now that doing this was because of vanity and pride, and I knew it was all right. I wanted to look good to myself, and then I would feel that I looked good to my husband. I also now know in my heart, that I feel this way because we were still in our honeymoon period. If we had been married for several years, I would not feel so insecure about my appearance.

In late April, I went back to Dr. Geoffrey for a follow-up visit. His nurse and medical assistant came in to chat with me before the doctor came in. I told Sabrina about the breast and how it was smaller, and that I could see and feel the implant. I also told her that my husband was afraid to touch it, believing that he would hurt me, somehow. We talked about our sexual problems and she was very supportive. She said that we had to re-learn how to be creative in our love-making.

Dr. Geoffrey came in and said that Sabrina told him a little about what was going on. He had me get down from the table and sit in front of him in a chair. He wanted to know if we were having sex and how it was going. He is the one person who I am comfortable with talking about our sex life. He then had me stand in front of him and he examined the breasts. He said that he could put a silicone implant in the right breast, but he did not want to touch the pocket of the implant right now. He said he could make an incision where the graft was and lift the breast up a little more. He would then have to reduce the left breast because it was larger, and doing this would make them more symmetrical.

He asked if I was all right with that and I told him that I was. I just needed for Wayne to be able to touch that breast so that I didn't feel so uncomfortable. I also told him that I thought wanting to have it done was vanity. He smiled and said that he was glad that it was vanity, because then I was not thinking about the cancer anymore. Then he smiled and said, "I know that you want more pictures taken." He said that he had to that because he was going to do more surgery. I told him I wanted fifty dollars for the pictures!

He took me down the hall and into the room with the blue drape. I struggled inside of myself once again to stand there with my chest exposed. I stood directly facing him, with my arms up in the air, then at a forty-five degree angle to the left, and then ninety degrees to the left. Then we repeated the process for the right side. Even though he had never made me feel uncomfortable, tears started to build up in my eyes. I stood there thinking that since I had done this numerous times before, I should be able to do it this time without crying. There I was, setting expectations for myself again!

He left the room so I could dress. He completed the paperwork so his office clerk could schedule the surgery. He gave me a hug and told me to keep him up-to-date about the book. He said that he gave the copy that I had given him to one of his patients with breast cancer, and told her that I was still completing it. She wanted to read the finished product. I told him that I would let him know when it was published. He smiled and said, "See, you have already helped one person."

Walking out to the car, I was excited that he felt my first book, *Surviving Breast Cancer,* would help someone. It was my purpose for writing it. Then I started thinking about more surgery. I was concerned again that with all the healing problems in the past, that there might be problems this time. I decided to relax and stay calm, knowing nothing was going to go wrong. This time the breasts would heal properly. I would look better to myself, and my husband would be able to touch me without being afraid. That fact, in itself, made me excited!

I called Wayne to see when he was coming home and he was already on his way. It was late, but I wanted to tell him about my appointment with Dr. Geoffrey. I explained what he had told me and then I told him that I would show him when he got home. I also told him that there would not be much discomfort, or pain, as Wayne refers to it. He was so happy that I would not have much pain. I did tell him that I did not ask how long I would have to be off work, and I was not going to ask.

My husband is a worrywart, as I have told you before. If there is nothing to worry about, he will find something. Our finances were something that he worried about all the time. I told him that we would be fine and I knew that I wouldn't be off work for more than a few days. He said that we would just have to save our pennies. I told him that I had to do this because I wanted to be perfect for him, and for me. I know that is my ego talking and that is all right. I am still young, we are newlyweds, and I want him to be able to touch my breast without being afraid.

I was crying and he told me not to cry. I was perfect to him and I needed to remember that he loves me for who I am, and not whether I had one or two breasts. Nor did it matter if one was not the same size as the other. It matters to me, though, and it's more important that I can accept my new body image.

I also told him that Dr. Geoffrey gave the incomplete version of my book to one of his patients with breast cancer. He was so excited. He felt that it was worthwhile to give it to her and that she was excited to read the completed version. I told him that I was going to make a copy for her and send it to him so that he could give it to her. He told me that he was proud of me, and admired me for all that I had been through. I reminded him that we had been through this together and we have shared this journey.

One of the things that I like about Dr. Geoffrey is that his patients are not breast cancer patients. They are 'patients with breast cancer.' I think that reflects his compassion and passion for the human being. He is a Michelangelo of the twenty-first century! I have so much respect and admiration for him. He stood by me and promised that he would see me through all this, and he has not let me down. He has always been there to listen and support me, and giving encouragement during my lowest moments. He shared my sadness, my frustrations, and my happiness. He also shares the excitement of my book and the web site.

I talked to one of my co-workers the following day, and told her what Dr. Geoffrey was going to do. She shook her head as I told my story, and said that I wasn't listening to my body. She wondered how much more I was going to put myself through. I told her that I needed Wayne to touch the breast. She said, "That is his problem! I can't support you on this one. You are going to have silicone when there is all the controversy about that, just because of your vanity?" I responded that maybe it is vanity, ego, and pride, but that I needed to have him touch my breast so that I didn't feel like a freak.

I started to cry because I was hurt that she had said that to me. This was someone who had stood by me, supported me, and whom I thought understood. I had to leave the office for awhile to be by myself. As I walked around the parking lot, I just breathed deeply. I thought about what she had said and realized that I was allowing those words to have an impact on me. It was creating negative energy. She is allowed to have her opinion and it does not have to be mine. This is happening to me. It is my breast, my body, and it is not just my husband's problem. It is ours! She has not been through this experience except as an onlooker. I love her dearly, but I had to let go of those words. Otherwise, it would eat me alive!

I made an appointment for the following week to see Dr. Geoffrey to talk about the silicone implants. I also told him about the anxiety I was having to go through another surgery. The appointment was for a Monday. On Sunday, the telephone rang and I recognized the voice immediately. It was Dr. Geoffrey. He was in the office looking at his schedule for the next day. He said that he was sorry but that he was going to be too busy to spend adequate time with me in the afternoon. He would be glad to meet with me at the office right then, or we could talk on the phone if I had the time. I told him that since he took the time to call me on a Sunday, I had time to speak with him.

I told him that I was concerned about having this surgery for vanity reasons He said, " I am glad that it is vanity because it means that you are no longer thinking about the cancer." We talked about the silicone implants and he said that now would be an appropriate time. He said the breasts will look better, and they will feel more normal. I would have the fullness that I don't have on the one side of the breast, and neither Wayne nor I would be able to see or feel the implant.

He also said that I would have to enroll in a study. He has a nurse dedicated to do all the paperwork for that, and it would allow us to stay in touch with each other. He wanted to see me on a regular basis. He knew that I missed seeing him because of all the support that he had given to me. His compassion for his patients and the passion for his work, reflects in the hearts and smiles, and the new body image of his patients.

He wanted to have more time to talk to me again about the implants and the surgery. He said he would have Bonnie reschedule an appointment for me and that he would give me more information on the silicone implants and spend time with me.

After we said goodbye, I was just amazed that he took the time on a Sunday to call me. He could have been like most physicians and had his office make the call, but he didn't! All I can say is 'wow!' He is someone whom I never want to lose contact with. He is an amazing person as well as an amazing surgeon.

I told my husband that Dr. Geoffrey called and I relayed our discussion. He, too, could not believe that he had called on a Sunday. He said that he understood why I wanted to have it done. He said that he would support me in my decision to go ahead with this. I told my husband, through tears, that I needed to do this, even if it was for vanity's sake. I was also doing this for him because we are still newlyweds and I wanted to be as perfect as possible. If this happened fifteen or twenty years from now, it may have been different, but right now, this is where I am at.

Two weeks had gone by and I realized that I wanted the revision done solely because of vanity. I knew that it was okay. I called and cancelled the appointment that I had rescheduled. Bonnie told me that he could do the surgery in late June, but I would need to come into the office to complete the silicone study paperwork. That appointment was scheduled for the end of May. She also thought that the nurse who does the tattooing could do that before surgery. She said she would give the nurse my records and have her call me. She thought it would be that day! I was excited! The nurse called and she said that it would be best to wait until the revision was done, so that the nipple would be in the right place. She said he may have to make changes on both sides and then it would be uneven. She said that she gave Bonnie some dates in July. She told me to call for an appointment one month after the surgery.

I was so disappointed when we were through talking, that I started to cry. There was a knot in my stomach, and I felt that the rug had been pulled out from under me. I realized, though, that I had immediately set an expectation and when it could not be met, I was let down. So I sat in my office, closed the door, and spent time in my safe place, relaxing. When I came back to the present, I was all right. The sadness and disappointment were gone, and I could go on with the work that I had to complete before I went home.

Through this process, I mentioned that my husband never spoke of how he felt, with the exception that he was afraid that he was going to lose me. It was Easter weekend, and we were talking about different things that had been happening in our lives. He expressed that he thought we were growing apart because our thought processes about things were becoming very different. He said that he was afraid that I did not love him anymore. I was hurt, but I stayed in control. I tried to reassure him. I told him that I do think differently, but I don't love him any less. In fact, I love him more than I ever did before! I told him that he had given me strength and courage to be a survivor. I explained that I no longer had the desire to waste precious energy worrying about things that I could not change. I no longer had the desire to be an over-achiever and advance my nursing career. I had found that it is more important to me to just be who I am, sharing and helping others. I was able to accept people for who they are and not for what they did or didn't do. I no longer placed judgment, and I have been able to place others in an "us" rather than "them" category. I think what I was trying to say was that I see everyone as part of my family—a family of the human race, and the family of God's people.

The other aspect of this is that we seldom have intimacy. Sex is a very important part of a relationship. I told him that I needed his help with restoring my ability to be stimulated. I could not do this by myself. I carefully told him that a couple of nights ago, he had gone to bed before me, and when I went to bed, I wanted to be intimate and he didn't. I explained to him that when I felt the desire that I needed for him to respond at that time, and not reject the idea of having sex. It would help me to be able to respond to him when he has the desire, and not have either one of us become frustrated or disappointed. I told him that we were feeding into both of our insecurities when we denied each other intimacy. I reminded him of the days when he would wake me at three or four in the morning and wanted to be intimate. I never denied him that pleasure, even if I was tired or just simply didn't want to participate. I now needed him to be able to do that for me. As a result of the chemotherapy, and the loss of my sex drive, when I do have the desire, we have to take advantage of that. It would restore my abilities to physically respond to him. I didn't want him to become frustrated because it would take longer to stimulate me in foreplay to bring back the excitement.

He said that he understood, but he could tell that I felt bad because I thought he had let me down. I explained to him that he had not done any such thing, and that we were both trying to get over our fears. He is afraid that he is going to hurt me, and I am afraid that he doesn't view me as attractive anymore. I told him that the more times that we try to be intimate and show just how much that we care and need each other, those fears will disappear. We could find that we will be able to resume our normal sex life and I would have the same desires as I had before.

I reminded him that he always says that I have been through a lot this past year. The problem with that is he never included himself in that picture. I always have to remind him that he has been on this journey, too. Even though we made an agreement with each other to be strong for one another, he was silently grieving, and he needed to start talking about his feelings and his anger. He repeatedly says that we will get through this together, but he does not express what he is feeling or thinking.

Traditions are hard to break. He is a Marine! In boot camp, they tore him down into feeling as though he was nothing, so they could build him back up and make him feel worthy of being a Marine. I smiled and told him that is one of the things that I love about him, but that on this journey, he needed to take off that "Marine hat" and be with me. We had to walk down this path hand-in-hand. He would have to share his thoughts and fears, so that we could move forward together. Not separately! We fight to survive differently and at different speeds, but we can do it together!

I think that he understood but was not ready to talk. I no longer have the fears I think that he has, and being a man, a marine, it makes him feel uncomfortable to talk about it. I love him more than I did the day that I married him. He has such a good soul. He now needs my strength and patience to help him through this.

It is April and I went back to work after surgery. I had made an appointment with the colon-rectal physician that the nurse practionner wanted me to see. I filled out the necessary paperwork and then waited for them to call me. I was taken into a room and was asked to provide a very brief medical history. Then I was told that the doctor's assistant would be in.

She came in and introduced herself. She asked a few questions and then took me to the scheduler. I was shocked. I wasn't going to see the physician! I am not used to this type of service and it totally took me by surprise. No examination, no introduction...nothing!

I thought to myself, that this is the surgeon that they highly recommended! There was a plaque on the waiting room wall that said he was elected as one of the top colon-rectal surgeons in Phoenix in 2003. The words "Big Deal" went through my mind! It didn't matter if he was the top surgeon if he wouldn't see new patients and treat them as patients. I felt like I was a steer waiting to be butchered. Walking out to my car, I felt disappointed. I thought to myself, this doctor is too busy to even meet a new patient, talk to me, find out what is going on, and understand why I was sent to him. Here I go again! No connection with a surgeon that I am entrusting my life and body to.

I thought about calling another surgeon but then I didn't know how long I would have to wait. As it was, I would already have to wait over a month to have this procedure done. I just wanted to get this over with and move forward. I knew that when I told my husband what happened he would be upset. He was having problems with his job and I didn't want to upset him. I realized, though, that I should not protect him that way and I needed his support as well. I would not get the support that I needed if I did not tell him what happened.

Turmoil continued in mid-summer of 2005. My heart sank to my toes one morning when I found a mass in my mouth. The "cancer worry" blew up in my mind with a force like that of a hurricane. I sat in the chair as tears welled up in my eyes. I made an appointment that morning to see the doctor. I was afraid to go, but I knew that I had to know the outcome.

I waited in the waiting area for what seemed like a lifetime. Finally, I was taken into the examining room and then had to wait some more. Sitting on the exam table, wringing my hands, tears would start to form. I told myself that I was a nurse and that I needed to stay in control. I could not, and would not, allow myself to panic before I had some answers. Even then, why should I think the worst? Would it do any good? Would it change the outcome? No! I told myself that what would be, would be. I had gotten this far without any major problems, and I could go the rest of the way! She came in, sat in front of me, and asked what was going on. She asked multiple questions about the mass and then completed an oral exam. She was not sure of the etiology of the mass. She suggested that I see a specialist and have it removed. She thought that removing it would be the best thing to do to eliminate my anxiety.

I called the specialist and made an appointment. Sitting in the waiting area, I thought, "Here I go again." Anxiety started to build up until I thought I would explode! I was so nervous, sitting there alone, that my hands perspired. I was taken back to an examining room and the surgeon came in right away. Sitting in front of me, she took a history and then completed an exam of my mouth, ears, nose, and neck. Everything was normal with the exception of the mass. She, too, was not certain of the etiology of the mass and felt that it needed to be removed and a biopsy done. Leaving the office, my heart felt like it was in my toes. I called my husband and told him what she had said. I could hear the anxiety and fear in his voice. He said, "This year is not going any better than last year." I had to agree with him this time. It seemed that we were being tested once again. The nurse in me took over once again, and I told him that we should not worry about it until we had some answers. Then, we would deal with it and the recommended follow-up.

That evening after dinner, I told my husband that I was going outside for awhile. I didn't tell him that I needed to be alone. I just wanted to think and go to my 'safe place.' I sat under a large tree that we have in the backyard and closed my eyes. I went to my safe place. It is a beautiful place with green grass, flowers, trees, a waterfall, and running water rushing over rocks, birds singing, and rays of sunlight touching my face. This is my place to allow myself to feel worthy, allowing the positive energy of God's gift of natural beauty to flow through me. It allows me to feel the that is within me to connect to my surroundings. I feel safe there, peaceful and serene. I am not sure how long I was there. It seemed endless. When I returned, I was at peace and I knew that I could handle the steps that needed to be taken next.

The following day, I called Bonnie and cancelled the breast reconstruction. I thought that it would be fruitless to have that done if this test came back positive for cancer. She understood and said that she would tell Dr. Geoffrey. She wanted me to call and let them know about the results. She said if I needed to see him, I should call. She told me that she would keep me in her prayers and they would re-schedule the surgery when I was ready.

The specialist nurse called and informed me the surgery would be the first of August. She gave me the place and time. The surgeon said that I would not need any pre-operative work since I had just seen the oncologist who had done a blood work-up. I e-mailed Bonnie and Dr. Geoffrey. I told them my scheduled surgery date and promised to call them with the results and to reschedule the breast revision.

In early August, on the night before my surgery, I didn't sleep well. Wayne tossed and turned but neither of us said a word. We were up early. Wayne did not want any breakfast. I could not eat or drink. When I brushed my teeth, I had such a desire to drink some water. My mouth and throat were so dry.

We left the house at 6:45 a.m., planning to arrive at the SurgiCenter by 7:00 a.m.. We drove there in silence. Wayne sighed and I asked him what was wrong. He said, "Nothing. I'm tired." I knew that he was worried about the surgery. When we arrived, I signed in, and we sat on a couch. It was so comfortable that we both were about to fall asleep when the nurse called my name. We were taken to the holding area. The nurse had given me a gown and I was told to change my clothes. She took my husband to the surgical cart where I was to go when I had finished.

I was not worried about the results. As we drove to the SurgiCenter, I prayed. I told God that I knew He was with me, giving me strength and courage. I knew that He was going to take care of me. I asked for the Angels of Healing and Protection to come to me and surround me with their white light of purity and protection. I envisioned their power and felt the warmth of their light surrounding me. I was filled with peace. (Later, I will tell you about someone who is a medium for healing and what she has done to help me).

She helped me onto the cart and covered me with a light blanket. She took my vital signs and then presented me with a consent form to sign. I would not have an IV because they were going to use a local anesthetic. After the nurse left, I told my husband that I thought it was silly that we had to come to the SurgiCenter for this if they were going to use a local.

Dr. Engles arrived and stood by the cart as I introduced her to Wayne. She looked over the paperwork and then asked what was wrong with my right arm. I reminded her that I had had a mastectomy. She had forgotten and apologized. I told her that it was all right because she had only seen me once prior to this. She asked if I wanted "not" to remember today. I smiled and told her that I didn't want to listen to their conversation while she was slicing my mouth. She smiled and then went to get the anesthesiologist. The nurse came back and started an IV in my left hand.

His name was Dr. Lee. He was very nice and said that he would give me some medication that would make me sleepy, and I would not remember a thing. I would wake up very easily and I would have a short stay in recovery. Then Dr. Lee and the surgery technician took me into the surgical suite. It was cold and the circulating nurse was standing by the table with all the surgical equipment. I was told to move over to the table. A blood pressure cuff was placed on my leg, and they placed me on a cardiac monitor. Dr. Engles came in and Dr. Lee gave me some medication. He told me it was going to burn. I remember the burning sensation as it started to travel up my vein, and I remember seeing a large syringe as he asked if I was sleepy.

The next thing that I remembered was waking up and Dr. Lee and Dr. Engles were talking to me. They were putting sutures in my mouth and telling me I was all done. I was then taken to recovery and given some juice. The nurse there was very kind and compassionate. I remembered him from the very first surgery that I had prior to the mastectomy. I told him that I recalled his voice and we then started talking. He located my husband and told him that I was awake and everything was fine. After about twenty minutes, I was getting dressed. The nurse helped me into the wheelchair and took me out to the waiting area to join my husband. Wayne retrieved the car and pulled up by the curb.

Dr. Engles told Wayne that she wanted to see me on Monday and that the mass looked like a mucus gland but she could not be definite. She sent the specimen to the pathology laboratory and the report would be back on Monday. I told Wayne that it was going to be negative, but even if it wasn't, we would deal with it then.

It was time to see Dr. Engles. I was not as anxious as I thought I would be. I was calm and peaceful. I was not worried about the biopsy report. In my heart, I knew that it was not malignant. I had placed my trust in God and His angels of healing. As the weeks had passed before the surgery, the mass was getting smaller.

I enjoyed the drive to the surgeon's office. The sun was shinning, with some clouds in the sky. The warmth of the sun today felt good. I walked up to the office building and went in. Going up the elevator, I said a quick prayer of thanks. I signed in and knew that I would have to wait for awhile because the waiting room was full. I read a couple of magazines and then my name was called. I followed the nurse to the exam room and sat in a chair waiting for Dr. Engles. She knocked and came in. Smiling, she asked how I was doing and told her that I was doing great. The swelling was going down, and my mouth was just sore, but not painful. I said that the pathology report was there but had not read it. In silence, she read it and then said, "It was just a blocked salivary gland."

She looked at the incision and said that it looked really good. I told her that two stitches had come out and she said that she had put some extra ones in there just in case that had happened. She stood up and said that she hoped that I didn't have to see her again, although she enjoyed meeting me. I shook her hand and said thank you.

As I drove away, I thanked God again for listening to me and for answering my prayers. I called my husband because I knew that he was anxious about the results. He was so happy when I told him. He said that he was worried that it might be more cancer. I told him that I understood that fear. I explained to him that the "cancer worry" would always be there for both of us and it would ebb like the tide.

On the drive home, I decided that I would wait until Friday's appointment with Dr. Geoffrey to tell him the results of the biopsy. I knew that it was time to have the breast revision done. I had to prepare myself for more pictures on Friday. It would not be easy once again for me, but I would be able to smile because I knew that this time it was elective, and not a medical necessity.

I waited to be taken into the exam room, and I felt myself getting uneasy about seeing Dr. Geoffrey. I could not for the life of me understand why. As I sat there, I took some slow deep breaths. As I started to calm down, it became apparent that subconsciously I remembered a statement that my friend had said to me about going through a breast revision. They were upset that I was going to put myself and my body through this again, all for vanity's sake. They felt that if my husband could not touch the breast, that it was his problem.

I reminded myself that was her opinion. I did not have to take it on as mine. Not being able to be intimate was our problem, not just his. Wayne's inability to touch the breast was not just his problem, but mine, because of the way that it made me feel about myself. If vanity is the reason I'm doing this, then it is all right!

My name was called and I was taken to an exam room and given a gown to change into. Dr. Geoffrey came in with a big smile, and hugged me. He had me stand down to look at the breasts. Since he was going to do surgery, he would need more pictures. I was taken to the blue room, as I call it because there is a blue drape that I had to stand in front of for the pictures. He had me stand in front of him again. Examining the right breast that is contracted, he said that the outer side was still a problem because the skin was thin. He asked how I felt about the left breast. It looked normal to me but he had me stand in front of the mirror. I stood there and I could barely look at myself. I wondered if he noticed that. I told him the left breast was fine. I just did not like to see and feel the implant on the right.

He had me stand in front of the blue drape. This time I not only had to stand facing him and to the side, but I had to bend over. It did not matter how many times I have done this, I was still uncomfortable and embarrassed. When he was done with the exam, I held the robe over my chest. He told me that it would take some work but he could give me the fullness where I had lost a lot of fat tissue. He told me he would raise it a bit. Once again, he said that I would have to see his nurse so she could enroll me in the silicone implant study program. I would need blood work done just prior to surgery. I asked if it could possibly be done before October, and he said that he would have Bonnie try, but he didn't know his schedule. He told me that Bonnie would call me with the date of my pre-operative appointment and the date for surgery.

In mid-September, I went for my pre-operative appointment with Dr. Geoffrey. For some reason, I was nervous. I kept asking myself why? I was going to do this so that I would feel better about myself. The hope was that my husband would be more comfortable touching me, and he would not be afraid to hurt me.

I sat in the waiting area flipping through a magazine, and not really looking at anything. They called my name, and I went into Dr. Geoffrey's office. The nurse went over the consent forms. There were so many forms for many different things! They all stated the same thing, but I felt my stomach sinking. I was getting scared because I did not understand what all these procedures were for. I wanted to talk to him because I wanted to see if he was going to be able to make the right breast as large as the left.

I sat there, signing the consents. I could hear his voice but I could not bring myself to ask if I could talk with him. I could not tell the nurse, that I, a nurse, did not understand all the procedures! Then Dr. Geoffrey came into his office. He smiled, sat down and looked up the latest pictures that he had taken of my breasts. He reviewed my chart and then told me that he would remove the scar tissue from the right side and place a silicone implant instead of saline. It was as if he knew my question without asking, because he said that he would make the right side as large as the left. Looking at the pictures, he said he would need to put more saline in the left side to raise it. He thought the silicone implant was the best thing to do. It would give the fullness that I was missing, and it would feel more like a normal breast.

I told him that I was going to be going back to work soon and I needed to know how long I would be off work. He told me two weeks. Two weeks! My heart was racing. He added that I probably could go back to work in a week. My heart sat in my stomach. Is the new employer going to be all right with me taking two weeks off after I had only been working for three weeks? I could not tell him that I would have to go back sooner. He would want me to take care of myself and would not want me to expose myself to any infection. He told me that I would have to be enrolled in a research study and they would allow us to stay in touch. He smiled because he knew how much I depended on him for his support.

I left the office knowing that I would feel better about how the breast would look and feel after the surgery was done. Right now, I had no feeling in my breast. It was just what I felt with my hand and what I could see that disturbed me. That is pure vanity, and it is all right! I was also concerned about starting a new job and requesting at least a week off. What was I going to do? Would I decide that I should just go back to work after three days since the surgery was scheduled for an early Friday morning? I pushed myself, setting expectations that I might not be able to meet again! I would have to sit and think this out. I needed to be calm, logical and realistic. Otherwise, I would get myself into physical and emotional trouble.

Once again it occurred to me why having this breast reconstruction was so important. The way I perceived myself in childhood development and the way I was treated by my peers influenced me more deeply than I realized. When I was in grade school, I was tall, even taller than most of the boys in my glass. I was well-endowed for my age, but not a popular girl. I was quiet and shy. The boys teased me about the size of my breasts, and called me names. It made me feel ashamed and embarrassed. That image stayed with me throughout my childhood development. It even carried over into my adult development. I recall telling you that even later, during my first marriage, I did not allow my husband to see me naked.

The revision was constantly on my mind Having the breast reconstructed was nothing more than for vanity! It was not about my husband at all. It was all about me, and how I perceived myself. I wanted to look as normal as possible for myself. It had nothing to do with him personally. He loves me whether I have one or two breasts, with or without matching nipples. This was about the little girl who was teased and made to feel unimportant in her childhood. It was about the little girl who had been ridiculed for being different than the rest of the popular girls. This was about my own insecurities of not feeling attractive. Once again, this showed me how much my physical appearance was part of our society's physical attraction for the male counterpart.

Vanity! Vanity! All is vanity! However, as Dr. Geoffrey and some of my closest friends have said, it is better that it is vanity. It showed that I was no longer thinking about the cancer. It was all right! I needed to be happy with how I looked. I needed to feel comfortable with my appearance to be able to love my physical image, which would allow me to love who I was on the inside more completely.

In another month, I would have the surgery done. I was in hopes that when I looked in the mirror I would like what I saw and would not feel uncomfortable. I would no longer search for who I was or where I was going. I would be able to expose those negative thoughts and beliefs and to see them for what they truly were—unsubstantial! It was important for me to think about new and positive thoughts. I would have to re-train myself over time so that I could change my heart. I would be a craftsman, so to speak, and I would create the person that I wanted to be in my vision. That would put a smile on my face. It was a potential and I felt full of positive energy!

Energy. Do you remember in school how you were taught about energy, potential and kinetic? Potential energy is that energy waiting to happen, and not until it's moving and active, do we see it in its kinetic state. Kinetic state is the reality. Wow! That means we can create reality (kinetic energy) with our thoughts and beliefs (potential energy). Imagine that! If we change our beliefs, we can change our behavior. If we change our behavior, we can change our life! We should NEVER underestimate the power of our beliefs!

Suddenly, I found myself having a lot of pain in my legs. It was so intense that I went to see the doctor. She told me she thought it was from the anti-estrogen medication I was on. She wanted me to call the oncologist because she thought he would possibly order a bone scan. She increased my Motrin and said that should help the pain. She told me to continue the walking exercises, and to use the Jacuzzi. She also wanted me to start having massages again.

I called the oncologist's office and left a message with his nurse. She returned the phone call and said that the oncologist wanted to see me. She gave me an appointment for two days later. I sat in the waiting area. It was crowded. Patients were there for chemotherapy. Women wearing caps on their heads brought back memories that I had not thought of for some time. I started to get anxious. I was concerned that he might think that this pain was from bone cancer.

I was called into the exam room and given a half gown to put on. The oncologist came into the room very quickly. He sat down and asked me a lot of questions. I told him about the pain. He said that it may be from the Arimadex and he would give me a sample of another medication. He said that If I felt better, I should call, and he would phone my pharmacy to give them a new prescription. He also said that he wanted to do a bone scan to be sure that the breast cancer was not spreading to the bone. He was 99.9% sure that it was the medication, but he wanted to alleviate any concern on both our parts.

He did an exam, and again he said that he was positive that it was just the medication. He gave me a hug, and said that I was going to be all right. Doing the scan was just preventative, but he wanted me to keep my appointment in November. He hugged me. It wasn't a "big" hug, but it was a hug which meant a lot to me. Although he had always shown interest and taken his time with me, this was the first time that he showed concern. He allowed me to know that he understood what I was going through. That felt good! Leaving the office, I suddenly felt that the scan would be normal.

It was the first part of October and I waited to have the breast revision done. However, the "cancer worry" rose like the tide waiting for the bone scan to be done. The morning I was to have it done, I was emotionally all right. I was positive that it was going to be fine.

I had the isotope injected, and as I sat there, I started to worry. What would the results be? What if it was positive? What would I do then? I left the office and drove to a local shop for a manicure. I wanted to do something to pamper myself while I waited to return for the scan.

I drove back to the imaging center, and had to wait for thirty minutes. It seemed to take forever. I was getting nervous, and I could not sit still. I was wringing my hands. They took me to the radiology room and asked me to lie on the table. The technician placed a pillow under my knees, and my arms were extended at my sides. The first part of the test would take forty minutes. Another forty minutes went by, and I was told to sit up and then I could use the bathroom. There were four more pictures to take. I sat on a stool and could see the monitor. When the first pictures were taken, I could see "hot spots." My heart sank. I felt like I was going deep into blackness. Tears started forming and I could not help it. I started to cry.

The technician asked if I was all right. I told her that I was a nurse and that I saw the hot spots. Suddenly, she interrupted me and reminded me that arthritis also shows up as hot spots. I told her that it was just frightening. She handed me some Kleenex and then said, "Don't lose it on me." "Lose it?" I asked. In a soft voice, I told her that I had every right to lose it. We had been through a lot this past year, and I wanted to stay healthy. I told her that I had so much to live for. I didn't want to start over with another diagnosis of cancer and have to go through radiation. I stood there with my hands over my face. I could not believe that she told me not to lose it! Most people do not know what to say, and I am sure that she did not really mean what she said. After that, she tried to keep me positive.

After the scan was completed, I waited in the lobby to make sure the pictures came out, so I did not have to make another appointment to retake them. As I waited, I closed my eyes and took some deep breaths. I had to relax and remember that whatever God had planned for me, He would be by my side to carry me through. The films were okay, and she escorted me to the front lobby. She told me that I would get the results from the oncologist on Friday. I thanked her and she told me not to worry. When I left, I wondered if she meant that it was not cancer.

The technicians that do the scans and the x-rays are educated in school and by the radiologists to read the exams. They were trained to recognize fractures and tumors so that they could bring concerns to the radiologists' attention when they read them. I am a nurse and I can recognize "hot spots," but I was not able to differentiate if the hot spots were from arthritis or cancer. While driving home, I took a deep breath and just asked God to be with me. I would accept whatever outcome laid ahead of me. I would continue to be thankful for all that I had, and the amount of time that I had left. I'd feel this way even if my time was short, or if the results came back positive for cancer. I knew that He had plans for me and if illness was part of it, it was okay. As I drove home, peace settled within me and I could smile and enjoy the extraordinary in the ordinary. The weather was beautiful, in the low 90s, the sun was shining bright, and I was breathing in and out. I knew that I had a family who loved me so much, and I could not ask for anything more than that!

I could not change the results of the scan. I had to put the "cancer worry" aside so that I could go on with my day. I reminded myself that we cannot change what happened yesterday because it is in the past, and we should not worry about tomorrow because it is the future, and we do not know what it holds. We only have today—the present. That is why it is called a gift. I had to use it wisely, and enjoy all that I had been given on this day. Tomorrow would take care of itself.

When I got home, I checked my e-mail. There it was! A friend sent me this wonderful "food for thought" piece which would ease my mind:

24 *Things to Always Remember*

1. Your presence is a present to the world.
2. You are unique and one of a kind.
3. Your life can be what you want it to be.
4. Take the days just one at a time.
5. Count your blessings, and not your troubles.
6. You will make it through whatever comes along.
7. Within you are so many answers.
8. Understand, have courage, be strong.
9. Do not put limits on yourself.
10. So many dreams are waiting to be realized.
11. Decisions are too important to leave to chance.
12. Reach for your peak, your goal and your prize.
13. Nothing wastes more energy than worrying.
14. The longer one carries a problem, the heavier it gets.
15. Do not take things too seriously.
16. Live a life of serenity, and not a life of regrets.
17. Remember that a little love goes a long way.
18. Remember that a lot....goes forever.
19. Remember that friendship is a wise investment.
20. Life's treasures are people together.
21. Realize that it is never too late.
22. Do ordinary things in an extraordinary way.
23. Have heart, and hope, and happiness.
24. Take the time to wish upon a star.

Was it coincidence that this was sent to me at just the right moment? I do not believe that anymore. My family and friends always seem to know when I need to hear from them. They are there with phone calls, e-mails, and cards at the moment that I need them the most. I believe that I have been able to connect to them spiritually. When I need them, they are there. They are one of the many blessings that I have in my life. They not only have left footprints on my heart, but they have touched my soul.

I read and reread the 24 Things to Remember several times. I was setting limits on myself by thinking that the results would be cancerous. I worried about something that I could not control. Therefore, I wasted a lot of unnecessary energy. I can only take one day at a time, and sometimes only a moment at a time, and tomorrow is another day to enjoy the extraordinary in the ordinary! I would not allow the unknown to weigh me down so that I could not enjoy the day, and my life. I did not have to regret what has happened to me, to us, this past year. It was all right to be fearful, but I needed not to allow that fear to control me. I am strong and have courage. I have faith that God is watching over me. Tomorrow will be a new day. Next week I will have surgery, and afterwards, I will feel better about myself. It's a good day!

The week went by rather quickly and now it was time to have the breast surgery. I have been very withdrawn this past week. When I am this quiet, it upsets Wayne tremendously. I have even been short with him unintentionally. We were sitting in the holding area waiting for Dr. Geoffrey, when Wayne suddenly asked me if this was worth it. He said that he didn't know how I was going to speak at the support group about accepting a new body image if I was going through all this because of my own vanity. It upset me tremendously. He did not understand the loss at all, which I have felt this past year. He could not comprehend that this was part of accepting my new body image.

I told him that initially I was having this done for him. I felt that it would help make him more comfortable to touch me, and I realized that he may never touch the breast. He got defensive and said that I had to understand that he was under a lot of stress trying to deal with all the surgeries, his surgeries, work, and his boss. The stress took away his desire and need for sex. I reminded him that he has only touched this breast five times and that I knew what stress he was under. I have shared that same amount of stress with him. I have just learned to let it go and let things take care of themselves.

We were quiet after that. I saw Dr. Geoffrey walking towards me and he smiled. He shook Wayne's hand and then pulled the privacy curtains around the cart.

Wayne got up. He told Wayne that he did not have to leave. I heard Wayne tell him that he wanted to wait outside. Dr. Geoffrey then stood by the cart and gave me a hug. It felt good and I started to relax about having the surgery. I had to stand beside the cart because he was going to sketch his masterpiece on my chest. He explained what he was going to do, and made sure that I had gotten the prescriptions filled that he had given to me four weeks ago.

We then waited for them to take me into the surgical suite. The surgery was an hour late. As they moved me into the suite, I saw Dr. Geoffrey standing at the far corner. They had me get on the surgical table and the nurses got me ready before I was put to sleep. I remember seeing Dr. Geoffrey standing beside me, and taking my hand. As I was falling asleep, I found my safe place and was at peace. I knew that I was loved, that I was worthy, and that I was safe.

I was pretty uncomfortable when I started to wake up in the recovery room. They gave me something for pain and I drank a glass of juice. It seemed like only minutes had passed when the nurse helped me get dressed. We were going out to the car, and I was glad to be going home. When we got home, I called and made an appointment for the next day. Then I called the oncologist's office because I had not heard from them regarding the bone scan results. The office nurse called me back and said that there was increased uptake in the thoracic spine area. Dr. Langford wanted me to have some x-rays taken, and she said I could just walk in to have them done. She also said she would fax the prescription in. She would not tell me anything else except that the results showed the increased uptake.

My heart sat in my stomach! I just went through this breast revision to be comfortable with myself and now there is the possibility that I have bone cancer! Whoa! Wait a minute, God, I told myself! You have taken me this far through recovery. Why are you testing me once again? I do not want to be a participant in this waiting game. I want the answers now. I specifically want to know what the oncologist and the radiologist saw on those films. The nurse in me just swooped up and took over all the emotions that I started to feel. I was not going to go down this path once again. Unfortunately, I didn't have a choice. I had to wait, and all I could do was to stay positive and remember that I cannot change what is meant to be. I had to accept whatever God handed me, and knew that if He brings it to me, He will get me through it.

I could not sleep that night. I kept thinking, "What if it is bone cancer?" There is no cure. Would I be able to go through radiation, and would I want to? I just started a new job! Would I lose it? How and what would I tell my sons? I knew they would not take it well. I knew that I couldn't protect them from their pain. I would have to tell them. I was scared! I had been climbing the mountain of recovery and now have I've lost my grip on the rope. I've fallen back into the valley below. I am filled with fear and anxiety. I find myself wanting to scream and shout at God for doing this to me again. Why am I being tested beyond my limits? What have I done or not done to have to walk this path?

In the morning, I found the following positive affirmation on a favorite web site; www.free-positive-thought.com: Life is full of blessings, and not all are seen. Today, I fully experience the blessings that are all around me.

Positive Visualization

In my mind's eye I see myself surrounded by the blessings of God. I feel and sense these blessings even though I may not recognize them overtly. I imagine myself opening my heart to receive all of the blessings sent to me. As I take a deep breath, I imagine myself allowing my blessings to fill my whole body, giving me strength, courage, and understanding. I say a prayer of gratitude for all the blessings and the special gifts given to me. I combine these images with joy and let them go, knowing that they will create the good things I am visualizing and thinking.

I took this thought and went outside to sit in the sun. Closing my eyes I took myself to my 'safe place.' Taking several deep breaths to relax, I started to feel myself become one with the positive energy surrounding me. I thanked God for all the blessings that He has given me in my life, even for this journey with breast cancer. I started to feel safe, worthy, and at peace. I knew that I was in God's arms and He was going to be with me. I thanked Him for this journey, and knew that there was a reason for me, for us, to travel this path. I will trust in His Almighty Power and Understanding. I will allow Him to bless me with whatever path He is taking me on, for I know that He will always be with me.

I imagined being surrounded by a white light, breathing in the white mist, and watching it encircle my body, cleansing me and leaving from my fingertips. I beckoned the Angels of Healing to come and remove all that is in my body that did not belong, and to make me healthy and happy NOW! I asked them to come now because otherwise, they will not know when to come. I don't know how long I was there, but when I brought myself back, I felt peaceful, content, and was able to smile. I knew that everything was going to be all right. Even if it wasn't, it would be all right.

I called one of my dear friends and left a message. She called me back. I told her what was happening and I started to cry. She said that she was not going to tell me not to worry, but that I needed to remember that I had this pain long before I was diagnosed with breast cancer. The oncologist was just making sure that I was all right. She said that she could not imagine how it must feel, but she had a good feeling that everything was going to be all right.

We talked for awhile, and she asked me to call her when I found out the results of the bone scan, even if I didn't learn the results of the x-ray. She said a prayer for me before we said goodbye, and I told her that I would call her when I found out something. I am so lucky to have a friend like her. She has always been there for me, laughed and cried with me. She has left footprints in my memory and touched my soul. We will be friends forever. It was a few hours later when I received a call from the doctor's office. They told me that both tests came back showing arthritis. Then she said, "I think you knew that."

I told her that I didn't know. She told me that Dr. Langford wanted to make sure that the pain was not due to bone cancer. I do not have pain in my neck, just in my legs. Without warning, I told her that even if I did think it was arthritis, what did it matter? Anyone who has been diagnosed with cancer will always worry that it will come back. They are there to let me know what the results of the tests are, to give support, and understand the emotional roller coaster I was on.

I could feel myself getting angry. I have little patience with those who work in a medical profession who have no patience or understanding for the feelings of others when they're waiting for test results. No matter what a professional thinks, it is important to those who are waiting to hear the good or bad news. They have not been on the other side of the medical chart, been threatened with a life-threatening disease, or faced their own mortality.

Later that evening, I suddenly realized that this year was nearly over. Christmas would be here in another two months. What struck me, was that by Christmas, I would be less than five months from being cancer-free for two years! I started dancing! I told my husband that I didn't ever think I would to say I am home free, but I will be able to celebrate each year with gusto!

A friend told me that if I stay positive and believe, that I will be all right. I know I will. I just need to take all the positive energy from nature and let it flow within myself. I need to see where I am going in this journey we call life, and then I will be able to take myself wherever it is that I want to go. Life's journey is a train ride. We get on, share part of the journey with those who we first fall in love with, then we come to mountains and valleys, and get off for awhile. We share those times with others who come into our life; sharing our train ride. We share our journey, our experiences, our laughing and our crying. We share our hopes and dreams, joys and sorrow. We learn and grow from each experience and from those who we share it with. Every person who comes into our life has a purpose. Sometimes we become aware of why they have come in, and sometimes we do not. When they have accomplished their mission in our life, they leave footprints in our memories, and sometimes touch our souls. The train ride begins again and we start another adventure.

I think it is fair to say that each stage of our lives is a train ride. It's an adventure in growth which matures into adulthood. Even as adults, we continue to learn. We share our experiences with those we love, and even those we sit by in the park when striking up a conversation. We listen to our children, grandchildren, friends, and co-workers, and we learn new thoughts and ideas from them. When our journey comes to an end, we celebrate life to its fullest! We take another train ride to meet up with those who we have left behind on our journey. We leave footprints in the memories of those we have shared ourselves with, and we touch the souls of some. We will live on in the hearts and memories of all those whom we met on our train ride through our life's journey.

I will celebrate every day. I will enjoy life, and all those who are around me. Life is wonderful and I have been given many blessings. Even being diagnosed with breast cancer has been a blessing, for it has allowed me to learn my own strength and courage. It has allowed me to rediscover myself and learn that each day is a gift. The Universe will take care of itself if we allow it. If we stay positive and believe with all our heart that we are all right, then we will be all right. I challenge you to stay strong and be of good courage. Believe that you are all right and learn that you are.

When I saw Dr. Geoffrey the day after surgery, I sat on the exam table and he removed the wrap and dressings. I was anxious about it, and worried that the tissue may have started to die. I held my head down so that he could not see that my eyes were closed. He said that there was no hematoma, which he was worried about and they looked really good. He explained what he had done. For the first time, looking at myself, I felt contentment and happiness about the appearance of my breasts. Even though they didn't look the same, there was fullness on the right side where the mastectomy had been done. They were swollen, but they appeared to be the same size. He took pictures with me sitting and then had me put on the bra that I had brought along, and he took some more pictures. He wanted to show other patients that they could look normal with clothing on.

Even though I know that Dr. Geoffrey understands the importance of looking normal in clothing, I am not sure than anyone can understand the impact of this abnormal appearance, looking at themselves in the mirror. It does have an impact when we see that our breasts are not the same in shape and size, or we see a flattened nipple, scars or discoloration. It reminds me every day, when I shower, and getting dressed, what has happened. I will be reminded every day.

We were watching television and there was something on that reminded him of Vietnam. I told him that I didn't know how it felt. I only know what he felt and what others had felt. I could not comprehend those feelings because I had not been there. I told him that he could not understand or fathom the impact of having breast cancer and going through a mastectomy because it did not happen to him. No one could fully understand because they had not been there. We share our emotions and thoughts with others and they think that they understand. They may tell you that they do, but do not let that fool you. THEY HAVE NO COMPREHENSION OF WHAT YOU FEEL! THEY DO NOT UNDERSTAND! They only know that it is a devastating experience! They know you are in emotional pain, but they cannot feel that pain.

This is why it is so important that you remember that when someone tells you they understand, or that they voice their opinions, saying it's just a boob, or they ask why are you putting yourself through another surgery, or they say that is your husband's problem, you must remember that it is their opinion and not yours. You do not have to take it on as your opinion. You have to do what is best for you! They are still your friends. They still care about you, and they care about how you feel, and what is happening to you. They don't understand the impact it has on you, and they certainly do not know how they would feel until they have been in your shoes!

The most important thing is for them to walk this journey with you. They must allow you to share your thoughts, fears, concerns, tears, and laughter with them. They need to be able to listen, to be supportive and to be compassionate. They need to share their love with you and let you know that they love you even more than they ever did. I have not fully understood as yet, why it is that we feel unworthy after we lose a breast or breasts. Maybe every woman doesn't feel this way, but I have felt that way, and I have to remind myself that I am worthy.

We cannot allow ourselves to lose our self-respect, our self-confidence, our self-esteem or our self-love. If we do, we will walk in the darkness of a storm that will never cease to exist. If we allow ourselves to stay in that darkness, we will eventually need professional help to find our way back. We are the stronger sex, ladies! I truly believe one of the things that makes us stronger is that we allow ourselves to talk about our emotions, and what we feel. Talking allows us to learn who we are and why we feel the way that we do. This is what sets us apart from others on this journey! We learn through this grieving process that there is more to life than what we have already experienced. We learn to enjoy the simplicity of life and living. Suddenly we realize that making a life is far more important that making a living. We can enjoy the extraordinary in the ordinary! We learn that giving to others is therapeutic for us to move forward on our journey. We can continue our life's train ride. We can enjoy it, and we can embrace it. We have learned that there is nothing worth worrying about in the sharp curves and corners of life, because the Universe will take care of itself. There is nothing more important to us than health, family and happiness.

I want to encourage you to be strong, and to be positive! Love yourself and do things for yourself. Work at rediscovering who you are. Yes, it is work! We may have to admit selfish thoughts or beliefs to ourselves, but it is a learning process, and our growth through adulthood. It is okay to be afraid, but use that fear to redirect your thought processes so you can understand the path you need to take to find the comfort and peace that you so desire. Learn to love yourself once again. You are not less of a woman than before. In fact, you are more! You are on the flight of new beginnings, of new life just as the butterfly begins its new life when it struggles out of its cocoon. So spread your wings and fly. Soar like an eagle! You will become the "wings beneath someone's feet!" Those feet may be your own, your family's, your friends, a stranger's, or an acquaintance in a support group. Share your unique self with the world, and you will be able to celebrate life!

I went to see Dr. Geoffrey for my follow-up visit after surgery. The past four weeks I have felt good about myself, and more comfortable with the way that I look. The breast is starting to feel normal to me even though it does not look the same. I realized one of the reasons that having this done was so important to me was because I was afraid that people would see what I saw. I was afraid that they would be able to tell through my clothing. With my hair growing, and looking normal with clothing on, I know that no one can see what has happened to me. Of course, Dr. Geoffrey wanted to take pictures. He said, "You know that you can't get out of here without taking some pictures"! I told him I knew that, as I picked up my clothes and headed to the room with the blue drape. I stood in front of the drape and he took the usual pictures. As I got dressed in the small dressing area he said that he wanted to take some pictures of me wearing my bra. I started to laugh. I don't know why I was laughing and I gave him a hug. Once again, I stood there and he took the pictures. He said his patients would appreciate seeing how they will appear normal.

I told him that I had just recently realized that looking normal in clothing was very important to me. Again, I had thought people would see what I saw when I looked in the mirror. He smiled and said that he knew that. I finally understood that all those pictures were for his patients with breast cancer. They would want to see that it's possible to look normal. It also gave him the chance to compare previous pictures while looking at the patient in person.

We continued to talk as I finished getting dressed. I wore my short-sleeved sweater and he told me that I looked great. Then he said that he wanted more pictures! He said that I was looking really healthy and good. He could see that my confidence was coming back. He reminded me to always keep a positive frame of mind, because the mind has such great power over the body.

While attending a conference in Orlando, Florida in November before Thanksgiving, I had a difficult time feeling comfortable around strangers without my husband with me. As I sat in my room one evening after dinner, I realized that I was afraid that someone would know I had breast cancer just by looking at me. Somewhere along this journey, I subconsciously did not want strangers to know just by looking at me, that I had had breast cancer and a mastectomy.

As I thought about it, I understood more why it was so important to me to have the revision done. I needed and wanted to look normal. The strange thing was that when I looked at myself, I saw only the image of myself without clothing on. I was afraid that it would show through my clothing. I forgot that people are not Superman with x-ray vision!

I knew then that Dr. Geoffrey was correct when he said that the fatigue may be related to depression. I was still healing, and working through the grief. My self-confidence and self-esteem needed nurturing and protection. I had not completely learned to love myself, nor had I fully accept my new body image.

I went to lunch with a former co-worker of mine whom I knew when working for hospice. She was retired now and enjoying her grandbabies. I don't believe that it was coincidence that we had lunch after I came back from Florida. We had not seen one another for three years, and it felt like it was just yesterday when we saw each other. We had a wonderful lunch together. We sat and talked about what we had been doing and then suddenly I told her that I was having a problem with my body image. I explained how I felt and she smiled. She said that if I looked around the room, probably half the women sitting there that had had a mastectomy. She looked into my eyes and said that she loved me for who I am on the inside, and not what she saw on the outside. Laughing, she said that if someone asked her what I looked like, she would not be able to tell them the color of my eyes or any other physical characteristic. She would be able to tell them about my personality only.

Isn't it amazing how God knows exactly what we need and when we need it? It is even more amazing that as we go through the grieving process, that we learn so much about ourselves and how to deal with the errors of our thought processes. The enjoyment of living is not where you have been, but learning from the past and looking ever forward!

I told Dr. Geoffrey that I had a new insurance provider now and that he was not listed as an approved physician. I asked him if I had any problems if I could still see him. He told me not to worry, and that he would figure something out. I just could not change physicians. He has been such an important part of my support system. He has shared my journey and helped me through some of the roughest times that I have had. He has been a "light of hope for me." He saw my fear and said that I could come to see him anytime. This was not the end of our relationship.

Chapter Two

In The Valley Is Where We Grow

It seems that the stressors and heartaches from health and financial problems in our lives come when we don't understand why, or how it could happen. We fall from the mountain of happiness and security into the valley of shadows in our lives. We find ourselves struggling to climb back up the mountain. As I look back at my life, I have been on top of the mountain of happiness several times, only to fall into the valley. I realized that when I climbed back up, I had learned something very valuable. In the valley is where we grow as individuals. We learn to have strength and courage. We learn resolve and understanding, humility and love.

Once again, I found myself in a valley. It was now June and we wanted to take our honeymoon at the end of August. I turned in a request for the dates that I would need off. We wanted to take an Alaskan Cruise. We had planned taking this cruise in 2004, but with all the surgeries and the chemotherapy, we were not able to do it.

I was not feeling very comfortable at work and the more I thought about it, the more I realized that I hadn't felt comfortable since I had gone back to work. It just wasn't the same. There was a lot of tension and stress in the office, and I felt isolated most of the time. Every day it was becoming more difficult to get up and go to work. It seemed that the days just dragged and I felt exhausted when I got home. Sometimes I was so tired that I sat in the chair and cried.

I talked to my husband about resigning, but we both felt that I needed to work until the end of the year when he could pick up health insurance at his employment. If we got health insurance from another company privately, we would pay outrageous premiums since we both had pre-existing conditions. Besides, I still needed surgery and he needed to have some surgery on his hand.

I remember it was early one morning when my supervisor called me into her office. She told me that she could not approve my time off. She told me that I had been off a lot and that I didn't have enough work-time invested for her to approve my request. I told her that I knew I didn't have enough paid time and wanted to take it without pay. Then she told me that she couldn't approve all this time off and not give anyone else time off. She asked me if we could cancel our trip and not lose any money and I was to let her know. She said she would talk to the administrator about letting me have the time. Two weeks passed and I had not heard anything after I had told her that we would lose too much money to cancel. Besides that, it was time to start making 'happy memories!'

I was really upset and I talked to one of my peers. She could not believe that she would not grant my honeymoon. I was angry. I felt that compassion for the staff was lost, which doesn't allow for the field staff to extend compassion to our patients and their families in a time of need. I called my husband. He was REALLY angry! Remember now, he is a marine. He told me to resign, and we would figure out what to do about insurance. I told him that I could get Cobra but that it would be really expensive. I thought we could cash in my 401K and pay off some of our bills so that we would not be financially stressed.

I turned in my resignation on a Friday and gave them six weeks to find a replacement. I was worried about my team because I knew that they would be really upset. If you recall, "Precious" or LouAnne, always said that I was the rock of the team. I kept them together, working together and when I wasn't there, they never knew what was going on. She always looked forward to my thought for the day, first thing in the morning.

I told the Peach Team on a Wednesday. There was sudden silence and I heard What?! in the background. I explained that I needed to take some time for myself, to make some happy memories. Some of them cried, and others were happy that I was going to do this, knowing I felt so much better. I told them that I would be back, maybe not as their supervisor, but I would be back. I laughed and asked, "So could you handle me just being another nurse on the team?" They thought that would be great!

During the second week after I tendered my resignation, things were not going well in the office. Tension was mounting and I was invisible to management. Knowing that type of behavior happens didn't make me feel any better, but it didn't make it appropriate. I was really hurt. I spoke with the corporate nurse and asked if it would be all right if I left now, since I had already resigned. She understood my need to leave and wished me all the happiness. She was not angry but was quite understanding of my need to start making memories. She said that she had a similar personal experience so she understood where I was and what I needed to do.

I spoke with Wayne and told him that I was leaving that day. He was in agreement. I resigned effective immediately, four weeks prior to my original last day to work. I said goodbye to all my co-workers. We all hugged and cried. They tried talking me out of leaving early, but I had to go. It was time!

Being a hospice nurse is a very rewarding career. My heart has been touched by so many wonderful people. The hospice family is filled with more passion and compassion for people than any other part of nursing. I will truly miss hospice and the people whom I have spent the past four years working with. It will always be part of my heart and soul.

I keep in touch with those whom I worked closely with. Occasionally, we meet for lunch. It feels good to be with them, to hear how things are going and what is happening in their personal lives. Life does go on! Eventually, we will lose touch. It's natural. For now, I enjoy the moments that I do get to spend with them to laugh and have a good time.

I am the type of person who likes to be busy and take care of problems. I see patients because I have a passion for nursing. Being a nurse is something that I always wanted to do since I was a little girl. Staying home presented a new style of living that I was not used to. It was difficult but I found that I was adjusting to it rather well. In fact, I was trying to figure out a way that I didn't have to work. The question that kept coming to mind, however, was how much do I tell the prospective employer if I looked for another job? I don't like deceiving people and not letting them know. Needing time off for appointments is not the way to make friends and influence people!

I found myself climbing back up the mountain to happiness when suddenly the valley appeared again. This time it was something totally different. Five years ago, after I had left long-term care as a Director of Nursing, I was named as one of the defendants in a wrongful death suit. It was now going to trial! I had to meet with a new attorney, and he said that I should be at the trial as much as possible. He was aware that I had been ill last year and he didn't want me to get overly stressed. He told me that I would hear horrible things about myself but that I should not let it bother me. I started thinking that maybe, just maybe, I was supposed to resign because I would have to spend the next four to six weeks tied up with this trial everyday. Could it be that God opened this door so that I could feel more comfortable not being at work, when I would have to spend time at this trial?

I went to court the day of opening statements and he was right. It was awful! I was angry and scared. The plaintiff's attorney was assassinating my character. He was questioning my integrity as a nurse and as a human being! I wanted to stand up and scream! I wasn't even the Director of Nursing when the patient had died. I did my very best when I was there, and I had not done anything wrong.

Every day, I sat there and listened to all the accusations. I had not shown any emotions of anger, or disbelief at what was being said. I would drive home totally exhausted. There was no energy left to get my husband's dinner. There were mornings when I didn't even hear the alarm go off when Wayne got up to get ready for work. I felt so guilty because he hadn't eaten a good breakfast.

Now we are into the fourth week, and I have gone through a metamorphosis. I went from being in a state of disbelief, to anger, wanting to be violent, and now to a state of acceptance. It was nothing more than a horse and buggy show. I couldn't change the outcome. The jury would base some of their decision on who they liked, the plaintiff and their attorney, or the defendants and their attorney. They had to listen to all the testimonies and decide the verdict. What a lesson in the court system this was! It was not at all like what we see on television. I went home now and I didn't even think about it. I dreaded going to court every morning. If I was not there a full day, our attorney filled me in every morning about what had happened during the afternoon session on the previous day. He prefaced it with, "You didn't miss anything!"

At the end of July, I had to be prepared to testify. I had been thinking about defending myself when I realized that I didn't need to do that. All I needed to do was answer the questions, and take the plaintiff's attorney back to the big picture. I was the Director of Nursing, the hand between the corporation and the facility staff. I looked at the overall structure, put procedures in place. I educated and taught on a regular basis to improve paper compliance. At the end of the day, I took full responsibility for the staff, and yes, I would occasionally miss a problem. However, working with the staff to ensure compliance, I was in hopes that the systems and education would bring it all together. I would not have done it any differently, and I had done nothing wrong. Once again, I realized that all I could do was be myself on the witness stand. I could not in any way change the course of events that had taken place. I would not be able to change the outcome. The jury would decide whom they liked and whom they believed. The decision was going to be in their hands. The end result, no matter who won, would end up in appeals court for another several years.

As it grew closer to the day when I would testify, I became increasingly more anxious. I didn't want to become too angry, because I cry when I am angry. If I was a juror, I think that if I saw the witness crying, I would think they were guilty. It had been difficult to read the jury's feelings. There was one juror, however, who appeared to be on the plaintiff's side. Every day I left the courthouse feeling very uneasy. There were two days when I walked back to the attorney's office after the day was over, because I felt so overwhelmed and disillusioned with the court system. The judge was inappropriate at times, and his decisions reflected that he was partial to the plaintiff.

The day I was to testify, our attorney told me to stay home in the morning, and to arrive at the office at noon. As I drove downtown, I prayed, giving thanks to God that He was with me. I asked for His angels to come and surround me with their white light, and protect me from being intimidated from the plaintiff's attorney. When I arrived, they bought lunch for me, but I was unable to eat. I was anxious but yet calm. I knew that I was going to do all right.

The others came from the courthouse, and we talked. Carol and I were on a roll! We reminded some of the attorney's assistants that we were menopausal women and the plaintiff's attorney needed to be prepared! We arrived at the courthouse about 1:15 p.m. As we walked into the courtroom, John, our attorney, turned around, smiled at me and rose from his chair. He took me off to the side and said that I looked very nice. He told me that I would impress the jury. He smiled and said that he was going to give me his best, and lead me where he wanted me to go. He wanted me to remember that we were just having a conversation, and that I needed to be interactive with the jury and him, when I answered his questions.

He started his direct examination. My voice was shaking at first and then I started to relax. I would look at the jury. I wanted to capture the attention of the juror who seemed to be consistently on the plaintiff's side. As the questioning continued, I realized that I had her audience. John had told the judge and the plaintiff's attorney that he would need three hours. However, he knew that he was not going to need that much time. It was a game! He had told me that he would be done in about one hour, and that the judge would call for a fifteen-minute break for a meeting. That would leave only enough time to cross-examine.

He started by having me explain my education and my past experience. He then took me to my marriage and wanted me to tell the jury that I had been diagnosed with breast cancer in 2004. Tears started to come to my eyes. I then had to tell them why I had missed some afternoons during the trial. As I explained all this to the jury, I saw the sympathy rise in the faces of all the jurors.

John then started talking about what I did when I arrived at the facility, and the systems I had put into place. The jurors were listening intently and taking notes. Even the judge was asking questions! I had calmed down, remembering that I had done nothing wrong during my tenure at that facility. I had done my best to improve the care. I was the resident advocate, and the facility advocate. John was done and it was now time for the cross-examination. I sat in the witness stand looking directly in the eyes of the attorney. I was not going to let this man know that I was scared out of my wits! In my mind, I said to him that I was going to make him look like the ambulance chaser that he is!

To my surprise he offered me a break, and the judge granted it. John took me to an empty courtroom and sat me down. He said that I would be just fine. I needed to listen to the questions and think before I answered. He was only going to have about two hours to cross-examine and then I would be done. John would then re-direct for damage control. Again, he said that he would give me his best, and that I should not worry. Court reconvened in fifteen minutes and I was on the stand. I waited to be treated as a hostile witness, but I wasn't. I realized that because John had me tell the jury about my experience with a life-threatening disease, that he couldn't because that would not look good to the jury. I listened to the questions, and if I didn't understand, I made him repeat it. John objected to several questions and the judge sustained them. The plaintiff's was upset. I knew then that I was making a good impression.

There was one question in particular that raised my dander! When I answered, I saw the plaintiff's attorney raise his head to look at me, and I saw the anger and astonishment in his face. I didn't give him the answer that he expected. His face became red and he started to get aggressive. Then he realized that he couldn't. I had nailed him! I had been looking at the jury and saw several jurors smile.

It was 4:40 p.m., and he said that he was done questioning me. I was totally taken off guard because John had said that at 4:50 p.m. he was going to remind the judge how much time the plaintiff had taken and wanted to re-direct. John, however, said that he had no further questions. Court was dismissed and would reconvene on Tuesday. The jury was excused and I left the witness stand.

With the jury out of the courtroom, John came over to me and said that I had done a great job! I started to cry because I thought at one point during the cross-examination that I had said too much, and that I had let my anger be seen. He placed his hands on my arms and told me that I was calm and there was no evidence of anger. He hugged me and said that he should hire me! Pam, his legal nurse assistant, came and put her arms around me. She also told me that I had done a great job and then asked if I was all right. I told her that I was. She asked again if I was sure. I told her that I was.

As I drove home, I told myself I was finished. I had done my best and now it was up to the jury to decide. The sad part of this is, no matter what, the plaintiffs would be rewarded a settlement. Just how much the settlement would be, would be decided by the jury. There was nothing that any of us could do to change that! I thanked God for being with me, and helping me get through the day.

The trial continued for another week. On a Friday, the plaintiff's attorney dismissed all charges against those who were named as defendants, including me. The charges remained against the facility. The following Tuesday, the jury would deliberate and hopefully by Wednesday, they would have made their decision. We would be out of town. I asked our attorney to call me and let me know the outcome. He was so excited that I was going to be able to 'get out of town,' and he said that he would call me and let me know.

I told him that I appreciated all that he did for me. I told him that he was one of those special people who cross our paths and leave footprints in our hearts. He was touched. We talked for awhile longer and he told me that he was glad that he got to meet me. He had wished it would have been under different circumstances. He thought I was a special person. Tears formed in my eyes. I told him that I would keep in touch. Again, I thanked him for his passion for defending his clients and for his compassion. He was very kind and understanding, helping me through this difficult ordeal! (I am sure that you would like to know the outcome. Well, the defendant's won! The plaintiffs were not awarded anything).

Several months passed, and I decided to try to go back to work. I was offered a management position with a home health agency. Even though I was excited, I was concerned. I was overcome with fatigue and continued to have pain in my legs. I awoke in the morning as tired as when I went to bed, because the pain didn't allow me to sleep through the night.

Starting orientation for this new position, I found that by 1:00 p.m. I had lost all my energy. I felt totally and completely drained. Some days, while driving home, I would have to stop to rest before I could continue the drive. Some nights, I was so exhausted that I went to bed at 7:00 p.m.

The weekend came and there would be so much to get done. I had no energy to complete those normal household chores that we have to do such as laundry, cleaning the house, and cleaning up the yard. I would start trimming the shrubs and plants and I would not be able to finish. It would lay there until the next weekend for me to pick up. I am sure that our neighbors were probably disgusted with the way our front yard looked. I appreciated the fact that no one said anything or complained.

I have been asking the Angels of Healing to come to me every night to remove everything that does not belong in my body. I wanted to feel happy and comfortable. I walked either in the morning or at night and used the hot tub as the physician had instructed, but nothing worked. The fatigue and the pain continued to get worse.

When I had seen Dr. Geoffrey for my post-operative visit after the reconstruction, I spoke to him about it. He was honest and said that it was not his area of expertise, but he knew that healing wounds took a lot of energy. He said that maybe I had some sub-clinical depression still remaining. He could not explain the leg pain, and suggested that I talk to my oncologist to see whether it may be the effects of the chemotherapy and the Arimidex that I was presently taking.

I was so exhausted that day when I saw him, but he made me smile and laugh. I could see in his face that he was happy that he could do that. He told me that I looked really good, that I was getting my confidence back, and that I needed to stay positive. He reminded me of the power that the mind has over the body.

The next morning, I wrote to many of my friends, telling them what was going on. I asked them to pray for me. I sent an e-mail to a friend who had helped me before. I truly believe that she has been given the "gift of healing" because she helped me when I had found the mass in my mouth. She wrote, "When you go to bed at night, lay your right leg over the edge of the bed, and drain all the toxins from your body. Watch it leave through your toes. In the morning, when I showered, I was told to cleanse myself. I should start with my head and imagine a white light, like a tornado, going all the way down to my feet. I should replace that light with the white light of healing from the Universe."

She is a special and gifted person. Her gifts are being studied at the University of Arizona in Tuscan and she was on A&E in October of this year. I was amazed how she had helped me before with reducing the size of the mass in my mouth. However, to actually see what she is able to do on television, strengthened my faith in the power of the Universe and its ability to heal.

Chapter Three

Amazing New Paths Appear

Hope is like a road in the country.
There never was a road,
But when many people walk on it,
The road comes into existence.

-Lin Yutang

When I went back to work 8 weeks following the mastectomy. I was so excited about starting. I was tired and going through chemotherapy, but I wanted to do it. It was better than staying at home thinking and worrying. I took my release back, and when I spoke to "the powers that be" I was told that I would spend my time auditing charts and teaching nurses how to document appropriately. I would not be allowed to have my team back. I was told that since the new patient care coordinator took over, he had provided them with stability.

At that moment, I knew I was in trouble. It was implied that when I was the patient care coordinator that the team was unstable. We had lost two nurses; one could not handle the driving and the other one moved to Texas. I had hired two more and they were in orientation. I was told before I left that when I came back to work, that I would have my team back. Now, I was told that I wouldn't.

I spent the next three months teaching and training. Then the opportunity arose to take my team back as the patient care coordinator. In September, I was allowed to have my team back but I was given instructions. I had to smile and no one was allowed to see if I was having a bad day. Not allowed to have a bad day was setting the tone for the next nine months.

Some days, I could not hide the way I felt. I was consumed with feeling alone, overwhelmed with fatigue, and I felt threatened. If I showed that I was having a bad day, I was afraid that I would lose my position as a supervisor. As the days passed into weeks and then months, the good days out-numbered the bad days. I think that people forget that once the treatment is over, the close observation by the physicians is when it becomes imperative that you have someone to talk with and share what you are feeling and thinking. After everything is done, now is the time that I needed them the most!

There were a few people who came to see me and kept me on the right track. They supported me and gave me encouragement. I mentioned Diana, LouAnne and Jan in my previous book. These wonderful women, with such beautiful souls, have always been there for me when I needed to talk, cry and be held. They always listened and keep me on track. They made me realize that I was the same person, but I had to learn to let myself grieve. They understand that this experience was hard and that nothing would ever be the same.

On one particular day, I found another small lump on the left breast. I told LouAnne and tears began to well up in both our eyes. She said, "I don't know what to say." I told her that there was nothing to say and we hugged one another. She asked me to call her when I had the results of the mammogram and ultrasound the following day. Before she left the office, she searched for me, hugged me, and kissed my cheek. She whispered in my ear to call her right away.

I got the results two days later and paged her. It was scar tissue that I was feeling and not a tumor. There was relief in her words when she paged me back. When she came to the office the next time, she had the most beautiful smile, and her eyes just sparkled. She gave me a very warm hug. She has been such great support for me. She tunes into my feelings and then leads the conversation to where she knows I need to go. She gave me insight into why I felt the way I did, without me knowing, until I thought about the conversation later. She lead me to find the answers I was searching for.

I went to work, put in a lot of long hours, and I always wore a smile. Due to that, people forgot what I had gone through. These wonderful people reminded me that I have to refresh everyone's memory that I was still grieving. They reminded me that I work long hours yet I always have a smile on my face, that I laugh, and enjoy joking. I have never looked like I had gone through chemotherapy. When I did have a bad day, it reminded them that I was still working through the grief, and that I was fighting to be a survivor.

For several months, I had been uncomfortable at work. I felt that I was being monitored to see if I could do my job. Close to the holidays, I was overwhelmed with fatigue and despair. I didn't know what to do, or where to turn. I wanted to run away and hide. My husband wanted to have a Christmas party and my sons were coming with their girlfriends. I didn't think that I would be able to handle it all. I was afraid, I suppose, that people would not see me as a person. I was afraid that my sons would not be able to handle how I looked at the time. One day at work, I was crying uncontrollably. I felt it was best for me to go home. I did not want my team to see me so upset.

When I returned to work the following day, my supervisor came into my office and closed the door.
She said, "This has to stop! I cannot have you crying and talking to the other PCC's. You are placing your problems on them and not allowing them to get their work done. They have their own problems to deal with."
I was shocked. I told her that sharing was part of surviving and being a survivor. The hospice and nursing philosophy was one of showing compassion. It allowed someone to share their feelings and emotions so they were able to cope. She also told me that my team was supporting me more that I was supporting them. She then told me she had to run a business. I told her that I would apologize to my peers and team. She quickly said that she didn't want that. I informed her that if people felt that way, then I did owe them an apology. From that moment on, I felt isolated.

The following day, I apologized to my peers for burdening them with my problems. They were dumbfounded! They told me that anytime that I needed to talk, to just get them. They did not want to be shut out. If we had to go to lunch so that I could talk, then that was what we would do. They explained to me that they were there to support me through the grieving process, and I was not taking them away from their work. At the next team meeting, I explained that I had been told that they were supporting me more than I was supporting them. I needed them to be truthful with me, and if they truly felt that way, then I needed to make a decision about staying or leaving. Mouths fell open and they could not believe what I told them. The nurses all said that I am there at all times to help them solve problems, answer their questions, and help with patient visits. The social workers said that I was the rock of the team. I provided them with stability and direction.

Fear with changing jobs was the ability to get health insurance. I didn't want to be without insurance if something happened to either my husband or myself. We both have pre-existing conditions and they may not cover any problems that could occur. I do know that most insurance companies want a letter stating there has been no separation in coverage, before they will continue coverage for pre-existing conditions.

My husband had surgery not long ago, and I had to take the day off to be with him. He had a bad reaction to the anesthesia, and the surgeon wanted me to stay home with him the next day. I had paged my supervisor but she didn't answer. So I assumed that the answer was no. I was uneasy about leaving my husband alone, but I feared that if I didn't go to work, that I would be disciplined. I went to work and when my supervisor arrived, she asked me why I was there. When I told her, she told me to go home and have the team page me if they needed anything.

I do not get upset over things at work like I used to. My priorities have changed. I do not have the energy or desire to go out and have fun with others. The things that used to make me laugh, I don't laugh at much, but I laugh at new and different things. They don't understand that I will forever cry about what has happened—the physical changes and the loss.

Working in hospice is difficult. I have completed two admissions to help the admitting nurses and one was a young woman with lung and bone cancer. LouAnne went with me because I knew that I would need support when we got through the admission. Surprisingly, I found that I was meant to see this patient, because she needed to know that it was all right to have a second opinion from an oncologist. LouAnne tuned into her feelings and took her right where she needed to go. I was then able to show her that what she was asking was reasonable. She needed to have her bone pain controlled. She wasn't ready for hospice, and we told her that only when she was ready should she do it. I hugged her as we left. I told her that I hoped that she could get her pain under control so she would feel more comfortable. She smiled and said that she hoped so, too.

On the way back to the office, I was in a whirlwind of thought. Tears ran down my face because I realized that that woman could be me in the future. I imagined sitting at a table and discussing hospice care with my husband. I knew that his heart would be broken and he would not want me to give up. I thought about my sons and how they would react. I realized that I would have a difficult time deciding that I did not want any more done. It would mean saying goodbye to those I loved the most.

I face my mortality everyday, and at that moment, I realize that whatever will be, will be. I should not think about something that I cannot control. It is the future and I do not know what it holds. I am living now! I am healthy and free of cancer! I smiled and decided that every moment that I have is a gift. I needed to enjoy the time that I have with my husband, family and friends. Those moments are a treasure and far more important than any one thing else in my life! I needed to give the best of myself to them and have a full and wonderful life.

The next morning, I had a message in my voicemail thanking me for being so kind and supportive. The family was appreciative for us coming and urging them to get a second opinion. It made me feel good. I realized again that I was meant to go, no matter how difficult it was for me. I knew exactly what she was feeling, and she needed to hear that it was all right from someone who had been where she was.

My supervisor asked me how it went and I told her it was difficult for me. She said that she was worried about that. I told her what happened and what they had needed. She told me that I was meant to go because I gave her a gift by being in the same position. She said that I needed to see that I could focus on the patients' needs and assist them with their fears and concerns. I thought about what she had said, and realized that maybe I do belong in hospice. Even though it is difficult for me right now, I understand how our patients feel and can more effectively guide them through the end-of life process. I have had the same fears, and have cried for the same reasons. I believe that because of my own experience, I am able to understand their feelings and guide them to reach the inner peace within them. Knowing and understanding what my family had felt throughout the past year, I have the ability, more than I did before, to provide the emotional support more effectively to the family members. I also help them find peace with the choices that their loved ones have made—to live and die in their home among their family.

As the months passed during this first year, I became increasingly more uncomfortable at work. I knew that I didn't want to work. As supervisors, we were told that we laughed too much, and we were not working enough. We were told that we could no longer go to lunch together. This put a bridge between us and didn't allow us to vent and share problems related to staff and finding solutions. We had been a tight-knit group and now we were being pulled apart by upper management.

I just wanted to make "happy memories" for my husband and family. The hassles of office life were no longer rewarding and had become more stressful than it ever before. The office was filled with tension that you could cut with a knife. Even the field staff didn't want to come into the office, because they said they could feel the tension. People seldom said hello to me anymore, or even asked how things on the team were going. This also made me feel uncomfortable. Not needing constant guidance should be considered an attribute and appreciated for making my superiors more comfortable. I was not afraid to confront anyone when it came to doing the right thing for our patients and staff.

My husband and I decided that we would make plans for a couple of trips. We had not taken our honeymoon yet, so we made reservations to take a cruise. We then decided that we would go to California in the fall and spend time with my two oldest sons. Then we would go to a banjo/fiddle festival that my son, Evan, coordinates. We booked a room in a bed and breakfast in Sacramento and another in Columbia. It was going to be such fun.

I often think that maybe I have caused my own sense of reality to feeling uncomfortable. I am not sure. Some people have told me that it is true. The same person who told me that I should not share my journey, or burden my co-workers, would then tell me that I was a wonderful patient care coordinator. It was a known fact that when there was a problem, I never hesitated and I did what needed to be done. She had wished the rest of my peers would follow my example. She told me that my team just loved me and would be devastated if I left. The kindness, intertwined with the negative, made me feel confused.

When I told my peers that I was leaving, they were sad, but they understood. My fear was that I would become invisible to upper management. I worried that they would make my life miserable. They said that they would take it upon themselves to make sure that I was always visible. I explained that I was going to be a volunteer for the Reach to Recovery Program. I told them that I wanted to work on my book, sit outside and enjoy the beauty of our backyard and I wanted to watch the weeds grow! I would allow myself to heal emotionally and spiritually.

The Reach to Recovery Program was developed by the American Cancer Society. It provides support for men and women who are starting their journey. It assists those in the midst of surgery and treatment, and helps those who are where I am now—fighting to become a survivor after the treatment is completed.

To me, it is a privilege to help others find comfort and peace within themselves following such a tragic event in their lives. To help them understand that what they feel is normal, and give them the support that they need to realize that they will find a new normal life, is my goal. They, in return, would give me the most wonderful gift of all—sharing their journey with me. At this moment, I cannot begin to comprehend the spiritual compassion, the passion of love that must flow through one helping a fellow human being, find him or herself again. I have known compassion and passion, and have assisted patients and their families through the end-of-life process. However, I believe that by supporting someone to find new meaning in life, making each day the best day of the rest of their lives, assisting with the meaning of being a survivor, would be a unique and moving experience.

After I was home for a week, nurses from other teams, spiritual care and bereavement coordinators began calling me at home to see if I was all right and what happened. I could not tell them how I felt I was treated, but I could tell them that my request for time off to go on our honeymoon had been denied. I realized that time with my husband and family was more important. I needed to take care of myself and enjoy my life now especially since I was feeling better physically. They showed so much compassion and understanding, that it brought me to tears. They were so supportive of my decision to make "happy memories."

After a week of just pampering myself, I felt so much better. During the first couple of days, I was sad because I missed the people whom I had worked closely with, and I missed everyone on my team. I made myself stay busy and I worked on the computer. I made cards and stationary, and worked with the production team for my first book, *Surviving Breast Cancer – There is a Child Within Us.*

I was no longer so tired that I didn't want to cook, so I prepared the meals every night for my husband. What a treat for him! We would eat dinner and then go outside to the pool. I couldn't go swimming at all last year and I was angry. This year, I hesitated getting in the pool because of my physical appearance. I am sure that I made it sound as if I was grossly deformed. I'm not! You cannot tell that there has been a change when I have clothes on. It is in my mind. I see the reconstructed breast, rather than seeing myself wearing normal clothing.

My husband has been getting into the pool for two weeks and I just started. I am learning to let myself go and just enjoy who I am, and how I look. Wayne tells me every morning and every evening that I am beautiful. That is so reassuring and comforting to me. He is so sweet. I call him my "Teddy Bear." He is such a sensitive man, who is so full of love and has such a beautiful soul. It is strange to me how my decisions can take me on a path that I was not expecting. Taking risks can lead to new opportunities and a brighter future. If I don't take some risks, I may never realize my hopes and dreams. I learn to dream the impossible and discover the possible.

After a couple months had gone by, another path appeared for me. I felt the realization of my hopes and dreams. I was asked to be a guest speaker for a local support group. The woman told me that she thought I had a wonderful story to tell, and the group that she was working with were now asking questions about body image and intimate relations. Since she believed that I knew exactly what they were feeling, she asked me to help them answer their questions.

I was so excited! This was exactly what I had prayed to happen. I wanted the opportunity to share my journey and to help others become survivor. I wanted to help them on their path or to rediscover themselves. I wanted them to learn, through me, that having breast cancer did not mean the end of their life, Rather, it was the beginning. This process of surviving is a life-long path. Each of us will struggle the rest of our lives, but life will not be a struggle. Why? Because we have learned to enjoy the extraordinary in the ordinary!

I wrote to my oncologist, telling him about my first book. When I saw him in September, I gave him a copy. He was very interested in it and also this book. For the first time, we discussed this journey and the journey of others. He offered his support by telling me that he was going to buy some books and give them to his breast cancer patients. He didn't want them to feel alone on their journey,. He wanted them to realize that there is life after being diagnosed with breast cancer.

I told him that I had written to several oncologists and plastic surgeons, in hopes that they would share my story with their patients. He said that he would talk to his colleges and encourage them to buy my book for their patients.

New paths were opening up for me. I visited my friends at my former employers, and they asked me to speak to the social workers at their meeting about my book. The administrator said that she would like to introduce the opportunity to the board of directors at the American Hospice and Palliative Care Organization to see if they would agree to let me speak at their next meeting in October. I was told that between 100-200 people would attend from various organizations! I was so pleased that she had offered this opportunity to me. I thanked her and told her that I would be happy to do that.

Chapter Four

Overwhelming Darkness Surrounds Me

It is only ten months since I had the mastectomy and I am now getting angry. I'm angry that this happened, angry that I cannot control my feelings, and angry that I am still so fatigued and do not have the energy to do the things that I like to do. I am angry that I do not have the desire to be intimate with my husband. I am angry that I have to work, and angry sometimes that I am still here. I have constant pain in my muscles and bones, and I cannot sleep through the night. I get angry with myself, because I cannot accept where I am in this grieving process, and I can't seem to move forward.

This anger is affecting my marriage. My husband does not know what to say or what to do. I find myself not wanting to talk, or else I say things that hurt his feelings. Then I get angry that I am taking this out on him. He stood by me, and was always there for me. He supported me. He would rather have me here and alive, then gone from his sight. My fear is that he will leave me because he doesn't know what to do, what to say, or how to help me. I have created a vicious circle!

This anger is destroying my self-confidence and my self-esteem. I look in the mirror and admittedly I tell that person in the mirror that I hate her. I don't like how she looks. I cannot seem to find my way back. I feel that I'm no longer an effective leader for my team at work. My mind wanders when I am there, and even at times I become bored. I don't want to go into the field and help the staff. I become angry because that is not who I am, or who I was. Before all this happened, I was out in the field helping my team with visits, doing supervisory visits, and I carried a small case load of patients. When there are problems that need a joint decision from the other supervisors, I don't offer my opinions. I am becoming complacent.

We, and I say we, because not only do I not have the desire for intimacy, but my husband is unable, also. He recently had surgery on his shoulder and he is unable to move it without discomfort. The nurse within me doesn't even come into play because I think that he should be able to move that shoulder. He is afraid to touch the right breast because he can feel and see the implant. When I bend over, the breast itself becomes very deformed looking. I understand that fear, but I still feel that he thinks that I look deformed and mutilated, which is the

69

reason why he doesn't want to touch it. I think about all the trouble that I have had with healing and getting it too look normal again, and now it looks abnormal.

This anger has taken away my spark for living, enjoying life and nursing. It has taken away everything that I have ever held dear to me. I no longer love myself which gave me the ability to love others, to see joy and happiness, and to enjoy the little pleasures of life. I used to enjoy working in the yard and now it is a chore. We don't have a sprinkler system and I have to water by hand. Being in the desert, it is a very time-consuming chore. It has to be done every morning, and it takes me more than an hour just to do the backyard.

I am angry that I haven't been able to clean out the pool. The creepy crawler device that rids the debris in the pool decided that it would break down and I haven't even taken it in to be fixed. The pool is a mess. I haven't even thought about getting in the pool at all. I used to clean it every week and spend the weekend in the pool just enjoying being in the water and getting tanned. I could not get in it at all last year. Now that I can, I do want to.

I have reread my journal and not once did I find that I ever felt angry. I didn't ask the question, "Why me?" So then why am I asking the question, "Why now?" We had only been married fifteen months when I was diagnosed with breast cancer.

I know there is always a reason for things to happen in our lives, but right now that reason or lesson is just beyond my understanding and comprehension. It frightens me. I feel that I have lost my way, and lost my ability to think and comprehend what is happening. I have lost what I am able to give to others, and to the ones whom I love. I feel that I have lost myself.

I haven't even used my rosary. It is not that I have lost faith in God, but I keep asking Him why now, and I don't get an answer. Maybe I'm not listening. I may be so angry that I cannot hear what it is that He is telling me. I have always had a strong belief and faith in God. I always listened and learned from His lessons, but now I just don't hear anything. I wonder if I am being impatient and trying to do this all alone.

Probably a support group would be an appropriate intervention right now, but I tried that before, and I started taking on everyone else's sadness. As a nurse, I wanted to fix their pain and I was trying to fix mine. I think now is the time for me to see a counselor, because I do not want to lose my husband. I also do not want to lose myself anymore than I have.

This is very frightening to me! I have always been in control, always had a goal, set expectations and strove to meet them. Now I have no control, no goals, and if I set expectations, then I can't meet them and I feel like a failure. I just keep compounding the problems. Sometimes I am not even sure what the problem is anymore. I am confused and lost, wandering in a place that is unknown to me. I am frightened!

While driving to work, I caught myself daydreaming. I didn't want to go to work. I was going in later, and wanting to leave earlier. I keep wondering if I should find something else to do. Maybe I need to be around people who will get well. Could I work somewhere that only required me to set up medications and do supervisory visits for home health aides? Maybe I could look into doing something totally different and unrelated to nursing, but nursing is all that I know how to do. Nursing is what I wanted to do since I was a little girl. Why would I want or even think of giving up something that I worked so hard at, and something that I have always been good at? Nursing has been the one thing that has always given me personal satisfaction because it allowed me to help someone else feel better.

The question that now comes to mind is why I have been unable to use everything that I have learned as a nurse to help myself to feel better? Am I so subjective that I have lost my perspective on what is happening, and what I am feeling? Am I capable of being objective?

As I write this, I know that I am not being objective because I am angry that my sons live so far away. They live in California and in Ohio. I need them closer to me. I am angry that I am no longer their rock of support, and that they have become mine. They are enjoying life, facing their own problems and I am not there to share that part of their lives. They call me to see how Wayne and I are doing, and I change the subject. I want to talk about what is happening in their lives so that I do not have to deal with my feelings. Lightening strikes and I realize I am doing exactly what my son, Brady did when we started this journey. He would change the subject and not talk about his feelings because he was angry.

I also know that if I told Wayne that I wanted them here, or to live closer, that he would not understand. He would feel that he was competing with them. He was an only child, raised by three women, and he sees them as "kids" and not young adults. He doesn't understand why I need them here. But then, maybe he does. I think that he is carrying around a lot of guilt feelings because when his mother was alive, his work took him away from home for months, many times out of the country. He wasn't able to spend a lot of time with her when her health was declining, and then she passed away. Even if I am not his mother, he wants to spend as much time with me and not share me. Being an only child, I do understand that.

I want my sons to live their lives and enjoy it. I don't want to be a burden to them. I love them so much but I really need them closer, or to be able to see them more than once a year. I don't want to be a burden to Wayne, either, and right now that is how I feel. It's like I have let them all down because I developed breast cancer. Now I cannot function the way I did before all this took place. I am no longer the strong and independent person I was.

I feel that I am alone, trying to find myself. I'm trying to understand what has happened and why. I am searching for someone who was and I cannot find her. This anger has left me frightened and confused. I need to understand who I am and where I am going. I need to find a purpose to all of this. This is a path that I have not traveled before and I need my family to help me. Yet, when they offer their help, I reject it. I push them away, and force myself to be alone. That is exactly the opposite of what I want. I am hurting them, especially Wayne. He doesn't understand and doesn't know what to say or do. I am angry and throwing words at him, but he doesn't know how to duck. He takes everything I say personally. It is not about him. It is about me. It is about suddenly having all the appointments, the monitoring and tests coming to a halt and having time to think about what has happened over the past year. I made promises that I would do really well with the surgery, and then multiple problems began happening. I'm hurting those I love the most, and that is the very last thing that I want to do. I just feel that I cannot help myself.

At work, we have a female counselor who comes in every month who we can talk to about what is happening in our personal lives. We can also voice our frustrations about work. She has been so much support to me. I told her about my anger . She reminded me that it was normal. She said that a lot of people become angry when all the surgeries and treatments are over. When I started this journey, I thought about just making it through the whole ordeal. Now I have time to think about what really happened.

She also knows my husband and said that I should tell him to duck, and to hold me when I am quiet or angry. She said that he should not take things personally. She reminded me that I had to reassure him that I love him. I told him what she said and he then understood. Since then, he has been ducking and holding me when I get quiet or start yelling.

I do not want to destroy my marriage. I would not be able to continue this struggle without my husband. If I would have been alone, I doubt that I would have done any of it. I would not have put myself through all this and suffered the way that my mother did. I realize, though, that my mothers' cancer was much worse than mine and I have not had to go through nearly what she did. She was strong, and determined that she would survive in the face of her immortality. I thought that I was strong and determined, but right now I feel weak and insecure.

I realize, too, that I am angry because I don't have a father here to support to me, and to hold me as his child and give me comfort. We have been estranged for nearly twenty-nine years and I have missed so much from that relationship. I am no longer angry that he left my mother when she needed him the most.
He didn't seem to care that he was taking away a vital part of my life, as well as my sister's. He wanted grandchildren and when he got them he didn't want any part of them. He robbed them and himself of a relationship. He took away the male figure in their lives who they could look up to and learn from. He lost the enjoyment of their growth into men, knowing that he played an important part.

It seems that everything that I was ever angry about, and now everything that has made me angry is coming to a head. I am overwhelmed with guilt and fear. I am afraid that I am a disappointment to all those whom I love because I am a disappointment to myself. I blame myself for what has happened. Why can't I accept that I did not ask for this? There is nothing that I did to get it. Today, I feel that the door to life has closed and I have no future. I am in darkness. I am not sure how to overcome it. How do I become a survivor when I fought so hard to make it this far? Suddenly, I'm returning to the very beginning of the journey.

I wonder if coming back to the beginning of the journey is the way to go forward again. Will it help me get rid of all the anger that was never felt and expressed? Can I rid myself of all the guilt that I have carried around in the knapsack on my back? Am I able to get rid of all the insecurities, self-doubt, vanity and pride, so that I can find who I am and where I am going? I long to find the inner peace and love for myself so that I can enjoy life and love others.

Maybe the purpose of going back to the beginning is to learn the circle of life, and to allow my sons to be my support. Maybe I need to make amends with my father, and learn to be dependent on others rather than being so independent. I want to learn how to love myself so that others can love me, and I can love them. I want to learn the meaning of "true love," which I know that I really do have with my husband, but I've been afraid to admit. I never thought that I deserved to have someone love me, or at least as much as my husband does.

Maybe this journey was brought to me to teach me how to forgive myself for all my past mistakes which I have regretted. We learn from mistakes as long as we listen to what we did and how it affected everyone around us. We grow from our mistakes. We learn who we are and what we want to be. We learn how we want to be treated and how to treat others. Maybe it is to teach me, and others, that there is another way to live life. We can find inner peace and contentment with who we are. We can learn how to deal with the outside energy that is around us, and we can make that energy positive.

Can we really take that outside energy and make ourselves feel the emotions that we have? Is it possible to stand outside of ourselves and look inside, telling ourselves that we don't want those negative feelings? Can we take the negative energy, turn it into positive energy, and guide our own destiny? Can we guide ourselves to have inner peace and contentment? Are there coincidences, or can we make things happen if we really think about it? Is life just fate, or can we really make things happen that we desire?

I remember an experience that I had many years ago when my sons were young. I had taken them to a wave pool about an hour from where we lived in Toledo. During our day there, I was in the pool when the waves started. They became violent, as if it was a sea during a storm. I was knocked off the raft. I flew up and then I came down hitting the water with my chest. My breath had been knocked out of me and I started to sink. I remember going down and seeing the turmoil on the surface of the water. The further I went down, the more silent it became, until suddenly, I was at peace. I was not afraid. I was filled with joy and happiness.

The next thing I knew, I was being pulled to the surface. I do not know by whom or by what. As I got closer to the surface, I could hear the sound of the waves and the noise from the kids in the pool. I reached the surface and took a deep breath.

It is that inner peace that I know that I need to find; that sense of joy and happiness. Otherwise, this anger is going to destroy me. I went outside and sat in the hot tub. It felt so relaxing. I closed my eyes, and I could hear all the thoughts that were in my mind. I imagined that I was sinking in that wave pool. The noise began to fade and I started reasoning about why I was angry. All the incidents that had occurred during my life flashed before me. I talked with those whom I was angry with. I had to let them know why. When I did that, I could let those thoughts and feelings go. There was no rationale for them. As I sank even further, I was able to be quiet, still, and could stop talking. The silence became deafening and I was filled with a sense of joy and peace.

In April of 2005 we went to see my son, Aaron in Toledo, Ohio. I also saw my father, whom I had not seen in nearly thirty years. Although it was difficult, it was something that I had to do so that I would have closure with that part of my past which had haunted me for years. I knew that we would not talk about what happened between the two of us, but it was all right. I needed to say I was sorry and that I loved him.

My Dad was never an affectionate person when we were kids. He never called me Deb, or Debbie. It was always Debra. Although we never had the relationship that I had always wanted, he was still my father and I loved him.

We drove to their home and I was quiet. I had a knot in my stomach. When we arrived, I sat in the car taking some deep breaths. Wayne told me that I didn't have to do this, but I did. I could not let him pass away without telling him I was sorry and that I loved him.

I could see the bed in the living room window as we walked up the sidewalk. The shadow of the man that I saw was not the man whom I remembered. I knocked on the door and I heard him say come in. As I opened the door, I saw my dad lying in a hospital bed. He looked frail and weak. He smiled and started to cry. I walked over to him, hugged him, and kissed his forehead. I stood beside the bed and he asked what had happened, since it had been nearly thirty years. I told him that I didn't know, but that I was here now.

Bonnie, his wife, came in from the kitchen. I walked up to her, said hello, and then I hugged her. Tears came to both our eyes. I introduced them to my husband. Wayne and I sat down and started talking. I could hear dad's chest rattle. His lungs were filling with fluid. I asked Bonnie if hospice had provided oxygen, and she told me the nurse was bringing it the following day. Dad said that he was pretty comfortable and not in much pain.

When my dad had retired, he followed in his dad's footsteps, designing and building clocks. He has made many beautiful clocks that were on the walls of the living room, dinning room, and hallway of their home. Bonnie got up from the sofa, and came back with a clock that Daddy had made for me, along with a throw that had been his dad's. The clock was in the shape of a cross. It was made of pine and "Lance Armstrong's Cancer Band...Be Strong "wrist band on it. I was so touched and humbled. I rose from the chair, and hugged and kissed by daddy's brow. I cried uncontrollably. He held me the best that he could. His arms were weakened from muscle wasting, and his breathing took all his strength.

When we were ready to leave, I did not want to go. I knew that he would not be with us much longer, and I had a sense of urgency to make up for all the lost time. I wanted to be there with him. I still had an underlying guilt nibbling away at me. Leaning over the bed rail, I said to him, "I love You, Daddy!"
He cried and touched my arm. I knew that he loved me without him saying the words.

I told Bonnie that I would call and come back soon. I gave her our phone number and told her to call us if there were any changes. She said that she would. We got outside and I started sobbing. It was uncontrollable. We put the clock and the throw in the truck, and I turned and held onto my husband. I looked back at the living room window and I could see my daddy. I wanted to run back in. I knew the next time that I would see him, he would be actively dying.

Driving back to my son's apartment, we were silent. When we arrived, Aaron and Mel were waiting for us. I wanted to talk to Aaron alone so we took a walk. None of my sons knew their grandfather. I told Aaron about our visit while tears ran down my face. He put his arm around me and I told him that when I come back, he should go with me. He agreed willingly. He said that our family was so small and most everyone had died. He only remembered going to see his grandma when she was ill.

I called my oldest son when we got back to Phoenix. I told him about our visit with his granddad. I started crying, and he told me that it would be okay. I told him that I was sorry that they did not get to know their grandfather and he told me not to be sorry. I told him that I would be going back and he said that he would go with me to give me support. I was touched by their compassion. They understood that after all these years of being estranged, that it was important for me to have closure. I needed them to be with me. They had also been hurt by the separation, but they understood my need to have closure with my daddy.

I found that I was not angry anymore but just scared. I was afraid that I would not be able to spend more time. We live so far apart and his life in this world was limited. It was a good visit. We cried together and told one another that we loved each other. I knew that he was not the father that I always wanted to have, but he was still my father and I loved him. There was no reason to be angry. I just needed to let him know that I loved him.

Although my daddy and I have reconciled the past so late, it is better done now than not at all. I cannot imagine the guilt that I would have to bear, if I had not gone to see him now that he was dying. I cannot imagine allowing him to pass from this life to the other without him knowing that I loved him unconditionally. I, too, needed to know that my daddy loved me.

Although it was difficult, I am happy that I went and I will go back before he passes. I want to be there with him when he does take that path to cross over to the other side. I found that even though I don't know Bonnie, his wife, I wanted to be there for her, too. It is not the nurse in me who wants to be there. It is the daughter who wants to be there, sitting by her parent, holding his hand, telling him that she loves him, and she will miss him. I want to tell him that he will always be with me.

After we were home from our visit, I wrote to Dad and Bonnie separately. I sent Dad pictures of his grandsons whom he has never seen. I wrote a story about each of them so that he would know them. I also told my dad that I did not really know what happened to us, but I loved him unconditionally and would be back to see him. Although I am sure that Bonnie knew I was not angry with her, I needed her to hear that I was happy that she loved my Dad and was taking care of him. I told her that she could call me anytime, and if she needed something or just needed to talk, I would be there for her. I would help her in the best ways that I could.

The anger and emptiness has faded now, and I feel a deep sense of sadness. I also feel a deep sense of relief. I have my father back. He is a different man than I ever knew. He is a man who shows his affection and true feelings, a father who shows his love for his daughter. Even though the reconciliation has come so very late, I know that it is never too late to share love and peace, and to share tears of sadness and happiness.

Once again, I am going to have to grieve a loss. I am going to lose my daddy that I just found after all these years. I have no memories of him since seeing him nearly twenty-nine years ago. I will only remember the shadow of the man that I saw on our visit the last months of his earthly life. He had stood six foot two, about 200 pounds of solid muscle, quiet, and with curly brown hair. He had a deep thunderous voice that made me freeze in my tracks when he was being stern, or when he was upset.

There will be a void in my heart for all the years lost, but I will be able to come to peace with it because I braved the rough water to meet him in his last days. I had let him know that I loved him. I knew that deep within myself, when I saw him, that he was waiting for my sister and I to visit him. It would not be long before I would receive a call from Bonnie telling me that he was declining rapidly.

After two weeks had passed, I had come home from work one evening, and there was a message from Bonnie. I called her back and she told me that my dad had started to actively die. I told her that I would be there either that night or the following day. She said there was nothing I could do. I told her that I needed to be there. She also told me that her friends drove by and found my sister's home. They had stopped and told her what was happening. She took the address but did not say whether she would go to see our dad.

I called Wayne and told him what was happening and that I needed to go home. I was crying, and couldn't control myself. I just found my father and now I was losing him again. Life is not fair, but I think that we now understand our loss and we do love one another.

I did not get there in time to see my father before he passed away. I was getting ready to go to the airport when Bonnie called and said that he had died. I asked it I could still come to see him. His wishes were for no showing or visitation, but she said she would make arrangements with the funeral home for me to have some time with him.

I was dressing to go and I felt so much despair. I was overwhelmed with grief. All the years that we had lost, and all the experiences of father and daughter were gone. However, the most important thing now is that we had reconciled. We were in a place that allowed us to forgive one another for all the hurt that we had caused for each other. Love and affection were both shared and now my daddy can rest in peace. I can grieve my loss of a parent and not be angry or resentful.

Aaron and Mel went with me to the funeral home. We were taken downstairs into another room and they brought his body out on a stretcher, leaving us alone. I was hesitant to go up to him. I touched his forehead, stroked it lightly, and looked into his face. Silently, I asked him to forgive me for being so stubborn, and for allowing both our fears to keep us apart all these years. I told him that I loved him and always would.

Aaron stood beside me and put his arm around me. I was crying. I told him how he had looked when he was younger, the man that I remembered. He said that he and Mel would leave me alone for a few minutes. When they left the room, they closed the door. I stood there, tears running down my face and I leaned over and held him. He felt cold, but there was warmth reaching into my soul. As I cried with my arms around him, my head lying on his chest, I could feel his arms around me and I could hear him tell me, in the voice of middle-age years, that it was all right. We both made mistakes, but he loved me, and he would be with me. He told me to be strong and enjoy life. At times, these spiritual experiences frighten me. However, as we left the funeral home, even though I was sad, I was happy. All that I ever wanted to know, even as a child, was that he loved me. I now know that he did.

I learned the connection between my inner self and the world around me. God is everywhere as well as within each of us. I was no longer angry about the events, or with the people in my past and present. I was no longer angry with myself. It was as if I had freed my ego allowing it to move elsewhere. I knew that I had to keep this feeling with me at all times. With all the thoughts about what was happening in my personal life, I knew there would be another storm that I would have to withstand. The question was, "How would I maintain that sense of peace and joy?"

In order to understand the feeling of peace that I felt when I was sinking in the wave pool, I decided to write about that experience and really give it some thought. So I closed my eyes, breathed deeply and slowly, while allowing myself to relax. I took myself back to that experience. I was sinking down into the water, the turmoil above fading, and there was silence. As I rose up through the levels of water, I came back to that place where I could see the turmoil. I realized that the peace that I felt was the connection between God and me. I knew that He was within me and outside of me. I had found how to get to the inner self, the spiritual self. I had to release my ego, because it always keeps me on the offense. It is just waiting for me to be offended. I had to accept myself and others as we are, and be aware of what was going on in the world. I had to give more of myself to others. I had to find that special something that makes me care deeply, and I had to put my time, energy and effort into helping make it better.

That "special something" was my inner self. I unknowingly allowed God's love to flow from me and into me from the surrounding world. I realized that was how and why I was able to release the anger that I had felt long ago about my relationship with my dad, and it helped to resolve our estranged relationship. It was how I knew that I loved my daddy unconditionally. I did not realize that it had happened until I had been diagnosed with breast cancer. I then knew that I had to let him know and began writing to him.

Now that a year has past since I was diagnosed, and I am still in a whirlwind of emotions, I can take this new understanding of peace and joy to the next level. I will be able to accept and be content with who I am. I will be able to work through the struggle to re-discover myself. I will have the strength and courage to fight to be a survivor!

Since I have written this all down, I have to admit that I feel more at peace. I know that I have a long ways to go, and I will need external help with this journey. I do sense that there is a way to find inner peace and contentment. I know that I can take this negative energy and turn it into positive energy. I can make my own destiny, and find that sacred person within myself. I will be able to love myself and accept this new body. I will eventually find that the person I was is still there. She has just taken on a different form, both physically and emotionally. I don't have to be afraid of who I am about to become. I will just be going to the next level in the circle of life.

It is difficult for me to imagine a world without desire. Can you? We want to create, and that gives us a desire! Most of us desire material things like big screen TV's, fancy cars, and advancement in our careers. I had those desires. I stress the word HAD! Now I desire to find the path to peace and harmony. I want to lead a simple life. Over the past year, I have walked down an unfamiliar path, not sure of where I was headed. What was to be my fate, my destiny? Could I control it? Could I determine my own destiny?

I have had several spiritual experiences as I have described to you. I have discussed what I have done to diminish the turmoil within myself. Now I find that I need to give myself permission to explore another path. I must allow my soul, the unseen energy within me, to take over so that I do not feel powerless over my life's circumstances.

I had to go back to my younger adult life where I remembered that my ego was totally in control. At that time, I was, as most others, concerned about my physical appearance and its ability to function. I recall working twelve to sixteen hours, and working on my days off. I was newly married. My body image and ability to work were vital for me to feel worthy. I needed constant approval to feel secure.

After my last son was born, I weighed 252 pounds. I went on a crash diet and when I had lost seventy pounds, I started to jog. As I increased my stamina, I could jog four miles, then six miles and finally eight. I ran 5K marathons. I lost over 100 pounds. This was one time in my life that I wished that my ego had not played a part. Through that experience, many mistakes were made. Even though I made mistakes that changed the course of my life, I now understand the path that I chose. Those choices, although having a negative impact, also has had a positive impact. I will not made the same wrong choices again.

As I got older, I continued to move through what I believed to be another stage that adults go through. That was when I decided that I wanted to advance in my career. Titles became important to me. I became certified in critical care nursing. I obtained a position in a highly respectable cardiovascular intensive care unit. I took it a step further. I changed the direction of my nursing career and became an Assistance Director of Nursing in a long term care rehabilitation center for three years. I was then promoted to Director of Nursing for another three years.

I spent those six years going to college to get a degree in gerontology. My sons were grown by that time. I had worked hard to have them receive an education in the catholic school system because I thought it would impress people. It would show that I was a "go-getter." I also wanted them to have a good education and to be successful in their chosen career paths.

When my oldest sons left home, I moved to Arizona with my youngest in 1997. I continued my career as a Director of Nursing, but I became disenchanted. I worked sixty to seventy hours a week and it was not making sense anymore. I no longer wanted to be an over-achiever. I had no life and I missed experiencing the really important part of my life. I was so busy making a living that I forgot how to live life.

Hospice care gave me a new purpose. I managed patients' care in conjunction with a physician. I provided comfort, education, and support to patients and their families through the end-of-life process. This support allowed their loved ones to die at home, with their family, surrounded by familiar sounds and smells. They died with comfort and dignity.

Hospice nurses have a gift to give our patients and their families. We accept them where they are in life, without passing judgment on where they have been and what they have done. We support them in their effort to provide comfort and dignity throughout the dying process. They give us a gift in return by sharing their life stories with us. I was able to serve others and felt grateful to be able to give to others on a spiritual level. I was starting to find an inner peace. The ego and drive to be a striving person seemed to fade from my sight.

I lost that inner peace that I had midway through the past year. I was on an unknown path, a journey which was foreign to me, in the sense that I had not traveled it myself. I had traveled it with my patients and their families, but I never truly knew what they were feeling until I was there. I was now on the other side of the medical chart. The nurse within me did not allow my emotions to surface in the beginning. I had to stay in control and logical. When I allowed myself to become an actual patient, my world went out of control. Every thought and emotion that I had kept in check, now came crashing in all at once.

I remember the "Little Red Engine That Could" story for children—what a good story for adults that need help to realize their potential. Remember the little red engine came to a mighty hill and said, "I think can, I think I can", and when he got to the top and was going down, he said, "I thought I could, I thought I could." What power that short story has! I combined that story with the first three letters of Cancer...CAN.

I found that so as I think, so shall it be! If I thought I was going to have a bad day, then I would have a bad day. I am going to have a good time at work. I will have a good time at work. So I decided if I wanted the invisible universal force to control me, then my thoughts, my reactions, and the circumstances I found myself in, would defeat me. I would have given up the ability or power to control myself, my responses, or my reactions to my surrounding environment. I needed to remember that everyone has a right to their opinions. We do not have to defend how we feel. We do not have to place judgment or let someone else control our emotions.

As I think back when my ego was obviously in control, I was in turmoil. I placed judgment and compared, trying to be right and the best. Now I am trying to find inner peace. When I am ready to act, or react, I sit back and ask myself if this is going to make me peaceful? If it is, I go for it. If not, I let it go!

I do not have to defend myself if I want to reach that level of a higher self having inner peace. Everyone has their own opinions and I refuse to get into a bullfight with anyone. I think that I am being drawn into an inner world, which is one where my soul is contained within my body. I want to reach a sense of spiritual peace and contentment. I want to leave my fears behind me. I am learning that my soul is limitless. Since we are made up of energy, we never really die. We are just ever-changing. We are part of all the external energy that makes up our life and the world. That includes people, animals, plants, the sun, moon, and the stars. I look at my body and break it down before conception and it is nothing but energy.

I believe what is happening for me is that I am learning to trust my heart because it uses intuition to recognize love, whereas the mind depends on having proof and logic for reasoning. I have been a fairly spiritual person for the past ten years, but I don't believe that I ever really connected the fact that God was within me, as well as in everything in the world that surrounds me.

Most of us are raised to think that God punishes us for our sins. He then becomes parental, an authoritarian and tyrant. So we develop a sense of untrustworthiness.

It is at that time that our ego grows and develops our external wants and desires. If you truly believe that God is within you and outside of you in all things, then you become more aware of all the beauty, and all the energy that surrounds you. We develop a divine trust, and that is where the inner peace comes from. We have allowed the love of all creation to flow between our external world and ourselves. We develop a trust in God. We lose our ego and become worthy.

I have chosen the path to find my inner spiritual self, which will allow me to find peace. I have to trust what my heart knows—love. I have to develop that place within myself where I can go and be alone, to build that awareness between the energy and myself that flows outside of me in the world. I will have to learn and trust that we are all one and of the same source of energy. I will have to let go of the ego and all its negativity to allow the positive energy to take center stage.

If I am right in my thoughts, what I will have achieved is empowerment. I will have control of the outside events because I will be able to trust my heart. My ego will be put on the shelf. My mind will no longer be looking for logic or reasoning. Every person, all of nature, and the Universe have connected energy, and it is this energy, created by the Creator, that will fill me with peace.

Sometimes I wonder if I am making the rediscovery of myself more difficult than it needs to be. Am I causing myself to be in turmoil when all I want is peace? Is of the turmoil that I feel the lack of self-confidence and self-esteem? What has caused me to lose those characteristics? Was it the cancer? Was it the mastectomy? Do I really think and feel that I am a different person because I lost a breast? Do I spend all my energy worrying about how my breast looks or doesn't look, and keep having the revisions done in an
attempt to have the past appearance of my breast back? I have to stop and ask myself, does it really matter anymore what that breast looks like?

For me to come to an appropriate conclusion, I would have to find my safe place and let go of all emotions. I would have to have conversations with those whom I know who would be honest with me. Then I could allow the energy to flow within, with the energy from my external world to find the answer and be at peace. With new faith in my spiritual self and God, I would make the right decision. I would no longer feel confused or in turmoil. I have found that I despise feeling unsure of myself. I question why I want to do something, if I am unsure of what the outcome will be.

On one particular weekend when my husband was working, I was sitting in the sun. It felt warm upon my face. I don't know how long I sat there with my eyes closed. I had turned on the waterfall so that I could hear the soothing sound of the water rushing across the rocks. I had emptied my mind of everything, including all the anger, the hurt, and the pain. I listened to myself breathing, slowly, in an out. I became relaxed and felt myself being filled with peace. It was as if I had let go of everything. It felt as if I was in another place and time. I felt my mother's angel surrounding me and I could hear her speaking to me. She was telling me that it was all right to be angry, confused and frightened but I didn't have to feel that way anymore.

She told me that I needed to take one day at a time, and if necessary, one moment at a time. Wayne was here to help me through this and he was not going to leave me. He loved me very much. My children, although far away, were thinking about me, and they would always be there with me. I raised them to be independent and to take care of themselves. It was okay for me to allow them to be the pillar of strength for me. It was their turn. I felt her touch my face, and tears began to roll down my cheeks. She told me that I was not lost. I was still the same person I was before I lost my breast. Our bodies do not make us who we are. It is that which lies within our hearts that makes us who we are.

She told me it was time for me to go forward and enjoy life again. It would not be the same, but I would find a new life. The old me that I thought was gone was still there, but I was learning new things about myself and I should not be afraid. I could not set expectations for myself that were too high to meet. I would only disappoint myself if I were not able to meet them. Taking one day at a time would allow me to succeed in finding the peace I searched for. It would allow me to find the happiness I was missing to fill my heart. I told her I missed her. She reminded me that she was always with me, looking over me, and she would not leave me.

There was a bright light that appeared and it was so peaceful and compelling. It was as if the sky opened up and she said it was time for her to go. I told her that I didn't want her to leave. I was crying. I have missed her so much. I wanted to go with her and she said that in time we would be together again, but now was not the time. There were things that I needed to do before it was time to be with her. I asked her what I was supposed to do. She only smiled and said that I would know. As she walked the path of that bright and peaceful light, my heart began to fill with peace and contentment. I was accepting this journey, and the path I have been forced to walk. I was filled with warmth. My heart began to slow down, and my breathing became deep and slow.

I was afraid to open my eyes for fear that all those emotions would come back. I didn't want to feel lost and angry, or out of control. However, as I sat there. I kept breathing deeply and finally opened my eyes. For the first time since I have been on this path of recovery, I saw the beauty that was in our backyard—all the flowers, the smell of the fruit blossoms, and I heard the birds singing a happy song. They are always happy, even when it is horrendously hot. They just take one moment at a time, feeding and taking care of their young, waiting for the night to come and cool them. In the morning, they start singing again because it is a new day.

This has been such a wonderful spiritual experience! My mother never looked so beautiful, healthy, or happy. I was moved by the event that had just taken place. I was shaking, but I was not afraid. I realized what I needed to do. I would take one day at a time, and even one moment at a time, if I needed to do that. I could not set expectations. I would just go through the course of the day, giving thanks that I was alive. I would remember that in the morning the sun was shining just for me. It would be a new day for me to learn, discover and enjoy. I could no longer try to go through this without giving all my feelings and emotions to God. I had to have patience and let Him take care of it in His own time, not mine! I didn't have to walk this path by myself. By being quiet, and not talking, I could reach down into the innermost part of myself and became one with God. I could feel His love and passion. I no longer desired to let my ego run my life.

I ran into the house because I wanted to find the poem Footprints. Margaret Fishback Powers described in her poem how I felt after I has seen my mother. It was through this experience I knew that I was not walking alone. I knew that my mother was there to give me strength and courage. Even when I was alone out to sea, or lost in the darkness, I was not alone. I realized that in all my trials and troublesome times in my life, the outcome always brought me to a better place. I didn't realize at the time it was God who was carrying me through those dark times. I didn't realize that it was God who gave me the answer to all those questions I had, and gave me the strength to go in the direction that I needed to go so that I could find the peace that I was searching for.

I looked back at the time I was taking a walk and it was getting dark. It wasn't the darkness of the evening that was frightening me. It was the emotional darkness that was so over powering. It was that darkness that was coming faster towards me as I walked. I had started to walk faster. I was breathing faster and harder. As the darkness was about to consume me, I realize at the moment, if I ran into the darkness there would be light on the other side. It had to be the fastest way to finding myself, making some sense of why this had happen. Running faster and faster, breathing harder, so hard that my chest started to hurt, I suddenly found myself in the light. Reading Footprints made me realize at that moment, in that troublesome time on my journey, it was God that took me through that darkness into the light.

I read and reread that poem almost everyday. It reminds me that I am not alone on this journey. It allows me to know that if God brought this to me, then He will bring me through it. I need to have faith and trust in Him. I will learn the lesson through this path that I am on, and there will be a reward. The reward is finding my spiritual self, and learning to give to others, to love others as they are, and not what they are not. The reward enables me to share this journey without expecting something in return. It allows me to help others who are presently on this journey to know that they are not alone. I want to help those who are fighting to survive find that inner fire within themselves.

I thought about what my mother had said: "I would know what I need to do." It was at that moment that I knew that I was to write about my journey. I would share my thoughts and feelings so that others would know that they were not alone. Knowing about my journey would give hope that they too could get through this. I have had a web page made for women and men, so they can share their stories with others. I include men because the spouses, partners, and sons are the forgotten ones. They, too, have to struggle to survive this journey that we are on. They, too, have had to bear the grief and fear. They have a story to tell so that they, too, can heal.

Chapter Five

Another Mountain

Bernice Ward

Can I climb just one more mountain?
I will try and make it one more time,
Sometimes it just seems impossible
But my hurts and fears, I'll leave behind.

God didn't say life would be easy.
He tells us to trust, He will be there,
So I will hold on and keep the faith,
And stay within, His tender loving care.

My climb has been long and painful
But I have trusted in my God for strength,
Each time I fall, He picks me up,
And wraps me again in His blanket of love.

My strength has failed, my body so tried
"God say," Child don't fear have faith,
Underneath you'll feel my wings as a pillow
Just rest in Me, "I will be your strength."

After months of concentrated attention, days mapped out by hours, I was suddenly dismissed and told to come back in three months. My health care team provided me the support that I didn't fully appreciate when everything was happening. When the weekly visits came to an end, and the whirlwind of all the surgeries and treatments stopped, is when the reality of the diagnosis of breast cancer really began to sink in. I was more scared after the treatment was over, than I had been before it started. I kept asking, "What now?"

Everyone concluded the disease was beaten and they were celebrating. I was expected to feel great, back to normal, and ready to get on with my life. Nothing could have been further from the truth! I was lost, like I was nowhere at all. I was scared the cancer would come back and wondered if the treatment had worked.

The separation anxiety took on new meaning. I felt I had lost my lifeline. I was not sure I could finish this journey on my own.

As the months have passed, there is a corner in my head for "cancer worry" that ebbs like the tide. It will always be there ready to expand again with any new unidentifiable sign or symptom. I realized this when I found a small mass on the left breast. The cancer worry became an elephant taking up all my thoughts, consuming my sleep and life. When the results of the mammogram came back negative, the elephant became a little mouse and the "cancer worry" shrank back to the corner reserved in my mind. I knew then, it would never go away.

Being able to share my thoughts and feelings with Diane, LouAnne and Jan became my lifeline after the treatment. They have guided me in a direction that has allowed me to soul-search, coming through this journey with a clear view of what matters most in my life. They allowed me to dwell in the darkness of my grief and helped me understand that grieving is a necessary part of the healing process, which allows my soul to heal. They helped me understand that nothing would ever be the same. All the supportive and compassionate care that I have given my patients in the past would now have a new meaning to me, because I have now been where they have been.

True friends are few and far between. People come into our lives with a purpose, and some leave when their job is done. I have found when there has been a purpose with meeting someone, they will always be there. It doesn't matter how many miles separate you, or how many years pass before you see one another again. You will meet up again, and start from where you left off . It's as if time and distance never existed. To my true friends I send this poem:

I'll Be Right There

Sometimes the waters get rough,
And it seems you might lose your way.
But whether in front, beside, or behind you,
I am with you every day.
So when it seems too much to handle,
Remember you can call my name.
I will always be right there for you,
Because I now you would do the same.

-Author Unknown

I have gotten rid of that backpack that carried all my insecurities, inhibitions, and guilt. I am taking some risks, and taking better care of myself. I refuse to worry about unimportant details.

Everything happens for a reason, so I just accept it. I am seeing the extraordinary in the ordinary! I have found my family is closer, and I refuse to take anything for granted. I will not waste time missing sights, smells, new flavors, sunsets and sunrises, watching the flowers grow and bloom, listening to the songs of the birds, music and writing. I have started to work on our backyard and found renewed strength and pleasure in cleaning up and refreshing my inner self with yard work. It is once again giving me inner peace, and reducing the stress and tension.

We went to Ohio to see my son and his family. I wanted to see my ex-husband's parents because they are now in their eighties and declining fairly rapidly. They have always treated me as their daughter, even though I was no longer a part of the family. Pop was taken to the hospital for an infection and we took mom home later after the visit. They plan to sell their home and move into an assisted living facility, which is something that they never wanted to do. However, mom cannot take care of Pop anymore. It is touching to see so much love between two people. They have been married nearly sixty years. It will be devastating to mom to have Pop die, and for my sons and their dad. I was glad that I could see them.

I have found that facing my past errors and mistakes, while forgiving myself and accepting others' opinions as theirs and not mine, that I can let those things go which I cannot control. I also have found that just spending fifteen minutes in the morning laughing is so stress relieving. It starts my day on a positive foot. I indulge myself. If I feel like eating dessert first, I do! I treat myself with a reward for making it through another day. If I need to talk, I do it. If I feel like crying, I cry. The biggest gift I found that I could give to myself is time—the gift to recovery.

When I went back to work, there were expectations that I could not meet. I had to listen to my body and the expectations had to be realistic for me, and no one else. I initially could not go to homes to see patients. I could not go out with a nurse to make visits. It was too much emotionally and it was physically too taxing. If I got fatigued and unable to concentrate, I would go home a little early and rest. Only a few of my co-workers knew of the fatigue and my emotional inability to see patients with my staff. If I was too tired to cook for my husband, then I would suggest going out for dinner. Or, I would ask him to pick something up.

Debbie Ziemann, RN

I would go to bed early because I was fatigued. However, I would arise at 4:00 a.m. to fix my husband's breakfast and to spend quality time with him. Then I would sit outside and watch the sunrise, listening to the birds sing their songs. I have a laughing session on the way home from work. I might be tired, but I could still make dinner and stay up a little longer with my husband.

Visualization was a helpful tool that I could use to bring a sense of peace and hope. It takes the positive energy around you in nature, and connects with the positive within us—our souls. It is spiritual meditation that calms the inner turmoil, to find its rightful place. Then, your hopes and dreams soon pull your heart gently to another world. I have provided you with a flower visualization exercise below. It is an easy exercise but it takes some practice. You must be able to empty your mind, sit in a comfortable chair, and allow yourself to become part of the chair. The surrounding noise will fade into nothingness as you fall deeper within yourself.

Flower Visualization:

*Picture yourself holding a small
bouquet of unopened flower buds. As
you breathe slowly in and out, the buds
begin to open. Do not breathe too quickly,
do not force the buds to open.
Little by little, as you relax and breathe,
the flowers will gradually become fully
opened. The tight, closed flower buds
will open to soft, brilliant petals. A
beautiful flower will appear from
seemingly nothing.
Relax your mind and body. Allow
your body to give and open, just like
the gentle opening of the flower buds.*

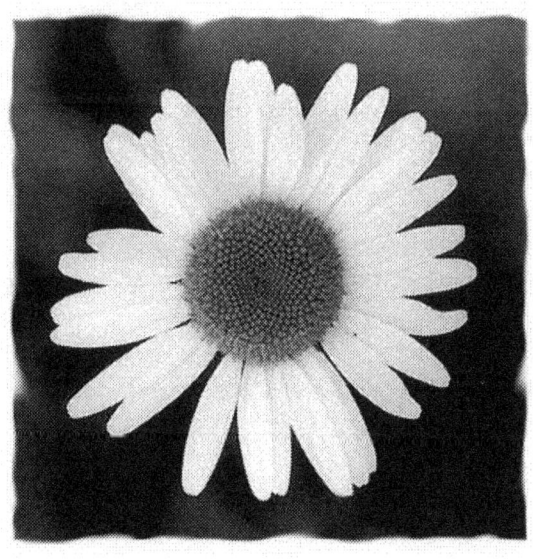

Keep practicing this method of relaxation when you feel yourself getting anxious and tight. If you feel lost and alone, stop and close your eyes. Do this simple exercise and you will find that when you return to the present moment, you will be re-energized and ready to continue the fight to survive.

I had to determine what my life would be beyond breast cancer. I am sure that it is different for everyone. I live one day at a time. I value each moment and every day that I have. I have chosen not to let this disease control me. I did not choose breast cancer. Instead of being afraid, I decided not to let the fear control me. I took charge of my future! I am not daring fate to plan vacations, retirement, and doing things I want with my family. There is hope that there will be years and years of a good life. Realizing it is not enough to say, "I'm alive." It is the quality of my life that counts. I try to worry as little as possible. It is okay to be who I am as long as I am not hurting anyone else in the process.

I told you earlier that I have chosen to have mammograms, breast ultrasounds and MRI's every six months. I know that by doing this, that elephant I described earlier, will fill up my space until the results are back, and then it will shrink. I realize that that is normal and it is just the "breast cancer worry" syndrome that rests in that reserved place in my mind. However, I do have some sense of peace knowing that if it does come back, it will be detected early. Anyone in this position has a choice to either adopt a bad attitude, allowing the disease to control them, or she can be positive and take control. We need to search for ways to have a productive, life-enhancing experience. We must accept ourselves for who we are, and how we look. We must pull our mind and body together, commanding a sense of well-being.

I want to live life my way. I want to set an example for my husband, family, friends and others. I need to manage my life to the very end. My family needs to see how I cope and manage my life. I believe that if they see me living a full and productive life, laughing through the tears, and enjoying every moment, that when the end does come, they will not feel empty inside. They will have learned from me how important it is to savor every moment, and make the best of every situation.

In the movie, "Tuesdays with Morrie," the professor tells his former student, "You do not know how to die until you know how to live." You have to live your life joyfully and fully. You must learn to sing as if no one is listening, dance as if no one is watching, laugh often and love much. You must enjoy every moment, and everyone around you. We have to learn to love ourselves so that we can love others, and then we will allow ourselves to be loved.

I think that this is a movie that everyone should watch. It gives you insight into living life to the fullest and helps you understand what enjoying life is about. I asked my husband to watch it a couple of years ago. We talked about the way Morrie viewed life and living, and saw that death and dying can be a beautiful experience. His perspective on living has gradually changed. He has started to enjoy the "little pleasures" of life. Every once in awhile, he reminds me that we have to stop and smell the roses!

Taking a walk meditation, I learned to listen to every breath that I took. As I concentrated on breathing I could smell the flowers, the wonderful bouquet of the roses along my walk. I learned to let go of the present and concentrate on someplace of peace and comfort. Have you ever stood on the beach of an ocean and listened to the sound of the waves on the shore? In my inner most thoughts I have been there. I have heard the ocean waves talking to me, realizing the beauty of the vast amount of water before me and how small I felt in comparison.

Every experience we encounter in our lives changes our thoughts process. We learn that we are ever changing, just as the ocean. We can take a beating and know that when the storm is over, there will be peace and comfort again. We always seem to bounce back, just as the waves flow back to the vastness of the ocean but only to return to the shore a new. I am being remolded with this experience of having had breast cancer. I am learning who I am, why I think and feel the way I do.

Although it is painful to be introspective, I realize that I am a product of my parents, grandparents, aunts and uncles. I think and feel the way I do because I learned from them how to react to situations. There were hurtful things that were said that left scars, and left me feeling insecure and self conscious about myself. I understand now that it is because of this I was having such a difficult time. It took me along time, but I forgave everyone that hurt me, and then I was able to forgive myself so that I could love myself. I could release all the negative thoughts I had about myself because I forgave those who had made me feel that way.

Jan came to see me the day I got home from one of the surgeries that I had, and we talked about my fear of finding more cancer when they removed my ovaries. We also talked about how I felt about not being able to respond to Wayne when he wanted to be intimate. Something that she said really began to sink in after she had left. She said that she knew in her heart and soul that I was healed. There was no more cancer. She told me that I needed to trust in my angels. They had guided me this far, and they were taking me to a new life. I am being guided to write and start a web page so that I can help others know that they are not alone.

She also said that Wayne and I need to make time to be intimate, and that without words, I need to take his hand and guide him to find the areas that give me pleasure. She said this is about me now, and that Wayne needs to help me and not be so stoic. She reminded me that intimacy is not just about having intercourse. It is about giving each other pleasure, and what goes on in a married couple's bedroom is for them and no one else. She told me not to be afraid of experimentation!

I thought to myself, here I am, fifty-two years old and she was right. I was afraid to experiment. I told her that the thing that was stopping me was the reconstructed breast, and that Wayne would not touch it. She told me that I needed to help Wayne get over that. I needed to do whatever it took to help him see that it is all right to touch it, and that I needed him to touch it. Even if I had no sensation, I needed him to touch that breast so that I knew that he was okay with it.

Shortly after Jan's visit, I checked my e-mail and found a message that I'd like to share with you below. It could not have come at a better time:

I thought about every phrase, and every word. I realized that God led me to this path and that His Angels are taking me to places unknown, where I can be of benefit to others through this experience. I think that maybe God saw in me, hidden from others, my insecurities and my low self-esteem. He decided that I needed to endure this journey in order to find my inner self and the strength that I really had—to find the inner peace that I was seeking.

I was living a life that had been taught to me: "more-is-better." This really starts when we are in school. We learn to pursue higher grades, additional diplomas and titles, along with promotions. If we are not pursuing, then we may feel guilt, shame, or think that we are being lazy and worthless or we might feel irresponsible. I needed to rid myself of this syndrome of more-is-better. I was finding the freedom to have the ability to choose rather than to accumulate. Only then would I be able to take that strength and this journey to truly help others.

I realized why writing has become exciting for me and why I really want to get out there so those who have been diagnosed with breast cancer, and those who will, have something that they can read. They will know where they are going and be able to understand that it is not the end of life. It is the beginning! Out of nowhere the thought of having a web page (www.survivngbreastcancer.com) for survivors to connect with others, and have some resources and support, became a reality.

Survivors, family members, and anyone will be able to go to the web site to find information that may help them. I've included medical resources, and links for books and poems. I have a message board where they can talk about their fears or problems. They will be encouraged to share their journey and become a survivor. They will learn to laugh through their tears. What I hope for most, is that they will learn that each day is a gift and each day is the best day of their life!

I have a sense within myself that I am now in control of my future. I envision what it is that I need and want to do. It seems that things just happen. Coincidences occur and suddenly it is as if the wheels start rolling and it happens. I envisioned having a web site and mentioned it to someone. Then suddenly, they introduced me to someone who was interested in creating the web site. I told them what I would like to have and be able to do, and it's done!

I am going to try to explain something. I have been meditating, and emptying my mind of thoughts so that I could look at myself on the inside. I search all my feelings and learned that I have been wasting a lot of time and energy with negative thoughts. I had fear, sadness and despair. When I worry or feel sad, I close my eyes and breathe deeply. I take myself to a place of safety and discover what I am worried about. I ask myself if it is worth it. If it isn't, and if I can't do anything about the situation, then I "let it go." Practicing this has brought me more peace and contentment than I have ever known.

Coping mechanisms are thoughts and behaviors that we use in specific situations, like when we have to change our daily routine or work schedule. How we cope is related, I suppose, to our personalities. For example, always expecting the best, or always expecting the worst, being shy, reserved, or outgoing. If we are committed and actively involved in coping, we will find meaning and importance in our lives.

After much thought, I believe there are several reasons that influence how we cope, and it depends upon: our own beliefs about cancer, the type of cancer and its stage, the chance of recovery, our individual coping abilities, our age, and our personalities. It also depends if we are negative or positive thinkers. Are we being honest with our emotions and feeling? Can we express them? That's vital. We cannot be judgmental about how we feel, which is normal, and we have to be willing to work through them.

Support groups are available for cancer patients. They are not for everyone. I tried a support group and what I found was that I was not able to handle other people's sad stories. I tried to deal with my own issues but hearing others' problems just made my sadness seem worse. Being a hospice nurse, I wanted to make them feel better and help them through the grieving process.

The support which was most beneficial for me was with friends and co-workers. Diana and LouAnne would sit with me. As I spoke, they would validate my feelings, and ask questions which allowed me to voice my fears and my feelings. Most importantly, they led me on a path to discover how to heal.

When I lost my breast, I did not feel whole, in spite of having a breast reconstructed immediately. Healing myself into feeling like a whole person has been very difficult. I had to transform my life, even in the face of death. I learned that controlling my emotional pain and personal suffering gave me hope for a future that possessed a life of quality. I know my friends and family love me. I found a burning desire to build new relationships with those who have been taken on this same journey.

Surviving cancer is a state of mind. I constantly read the following statement every morning to start my day, because survivorship is a long process. I need to remind myself what it is to be a survivor:

Traits of a Survivor

Being a victim is a state of mind dictated by others.
A Survivor dictates their own state of mind!
A victim fears the moments of grief,
A Survivor welcomes those moments!
A victim knows about feeling down and tries to stay
up.
A Survivor knows that feeling down is okay!
A victim tries hard to hide the tears.
A Survivor never leaves home without Kleenex!
A victim struggles to maintain a state of normalcy.
A Survivor knows normal no longer exists!
A victim gets caught in isolation.
A Survivor reaches out when they need to!
A victim is afraid they in time will forget.
A Survivor knows they never will!
A victim sometimes feels guilty laughing.
A survivor laughs through their tears!
A victim tries at times to block out the memories.
A Survivor embraces memories of all kinds!
A victim wants someone to cure their grief.
A Survivor just wants someone to share their
journey!
A victim struggles to get over their grief.
A Survivor fights to get through it!
A victim tries to get on with their life.
A Survivor lives their life knowing nothing will ever
be the same!

A victim says, "Oh, I'm okay," and then secretly
cries.
A Survivor openly cries, and says, "I'm Okay!"

This process of our healing is remembering who we are, and taking risks that we would not have done if we had not be forced to face our mortality. When I look in the mirror, the reflection is that of the new physical changes that have taken place. Who I truly am within has not changed. I just thought I did, but maybe to some extent, I have. What I now see in the mirror's reflection is that I have developed a special uniqueness in the capacity to love, to experience life, and to share my journey with those who have taken this same journey.

I have found a new path to a productive life. It is filled with a strength I did not know I possessed. I have a willingness to take risks, and the desire to enjoy what I can touch, hear, see, and smell. I want to share the love that is within me.

I am no longer so uncomfortable going out in public without a wig. My hair is growing and although it is short and curly, I accept it. I see people looking at me and I wonder what they are thinking or saying to one another. Sometimes, they look at me and laugh. I walked up to a couple of young girls who looked at me and were laughing one day. I told them although my hair may look funny to them, they did not appreciate why my hair looks as it does. It was not by choice. I told them that this was my "chemo hair." I encouraged them to think before they laughed at women with hair this short, because one day they may be in this same position or it may happen to their mother or grandmother. They apologized and I accepted their apology. I smiled and hugged them both. I felt better! People laugh because they are ignorant and have a lack of understanding.

I found the following poem on the Internet, and it helped put my thoughts and feelings into perspective:

Risk

To laugh is to risk appearing the fool.
To weep is to risk appearing sentimental.
To reach out for another is to risk involvement.
To expose feelings is to risk exposing your true self.
To play your idea, your dreams before the crowd
is to risk their loss.
To love is to risk not being loved in return.
To love is to risk dying.
To hope is to risk despair.
To try is to risk failure.
But risk must be taken, because the greatest hazard
in

Life is to risk nothing.
The person who risks nothing, does nothing, has
Nothing and is nothing.
He may avoid suffering and sorrow, but he simply
Cannot learn, feel, change, grow, and love.
Chained by his certitudes, he is a slave.
He has forfeited freedom.
Only a person who risks, is free.

Life is a risk, and how we choose to live determines what we receive. We have to be able to love ourselves, share that loving nature with others, and face the suffering and hurt, to grow and learn. We have to allow ourselves to feel all the energy that is within us and that which surrounds us.

Later on in the year when my hair was getting longer, I was outside and there was a strong breeze. I could feel the wind moving my hair. I got so excited to think that it was getting long enough to have the winds blow my hair. I found myself standing up with my arms reaching to the sky. I began swinging around in circles, smiling and saying thank you. I decided I would never get my hair cut again. It may be very curly but it is going to be long once again.

I have found that I am saying whatever I need to say or think. I try to do it tactfully so as not to hurt anyone's feelings. I am sure that I may offend some people. I suppose that it is happening so spontaneously because life is too short not to be heard. Maybe it is just because of this journey that I have taken.

This disease is not good or bad, but I have chosen to make it a gift! I am not happy about having had breast cancer, but it has redirected my life. Cancer in its own way has been a blessing because I have learned so much about myself and others. I have learned how to handle life's situations better, how to speak about my feelings, how to listen, and I appreciate others' thoughts and feelings. I have thrown away all the junk in that emotional backpack that I wore. I am learning to be content and committed to living each day to its fullest.

Cancer has changed my whole outlook on life. I now live day-to-day and enjoy each moment. I choose to be reborn. I am grateful to be alive, and I'm learning to live. I work at not measuring my life as it was or wished it to be, but how wonderful it is today. Each day is a splendid, unforgettable miracle, and a gift for me to savor and fully enjoy.

For me, it is vital to express all my feelings, including the unpleasant ones, because once they are all out in the open, they lose their power over me. They cannot tie me up in knots any longer! I think letting them out is a live message to my body saying that this is a fighting spirit. Keeping a positive attitude somehow must communicate to the brain a type of meaningful message. We take control and do not allow the disease to consume us.

Maintaining a positive attitude, arousing our feelings with the touch of someone's hand, appreciating the smell of flowers, the beauty of a sunrise or sunset, the music of singing birds, the calming sound of spring water running past and over rocks are life-enhancing experiences that allow us to enjoy life and living. We use the inner energy within us, and somehow it has a physiological effect on our bodies.

I relate this to pet therapy in long-term care. When our dementia patients were agitated, we would take them to pet therapy and amazingly they would calm down. They would sit for a half hour or more, gently and tenderly petting a dog or cat. They would become more alert and their facial expressions revealed love and peace.

When I enjoy the "little pleasures" of life and the beauty in each moment, that feelings promotes a sense of well-being. It fills my heart and spirit with peace. I am learning to listen to myself. It is not selfish. It is self-love and self-esteem which allows me the ability to heal. I can find my way back to the world in which I now live.

I think that Eleanor Roosevelt said it well, when she said, "You gain strength, courage and confidence by every experience in which you really stop to look fear in the face. You are able to say to yourself, 'I have lived through this…I can take the next thing that comes along.' You must do the thing you think you cannot do."

Chapter Six

Discover The Limits of the Possible

If God Brings Me To It, He Will Bring Me Through It!

In "Broken Dreams" by Lauretta Burns, she gives us the reason why we have such a difficult time healing. When we give our shattered hopes, dreams and our life to god, we must leave it to Him to work His miracles alone, in His own time.

There were times on this journey that it was very difficult for me to do that. I wanted things to be "fixed" yesterday! I wasn't letting go and I was trying in my own way to make things better, or make them right. When I was able to 'let go' and give the problems to God, the power of the Universe, my hopes, dreams and my life started to come together. I saw myself as a caterpillar transforming into a beautiful butterfly. It was then that I knew I was healing and I was going to begin a new life, with vision, hope, and all the beauty around. I was filled with gratitude for having another day to experience, learn and to grow. I was able to be thankful for what I did have, and not dwell on what I had lost. I became grateful to have had this experience!

If I had not traveled this path, I would never have learned of the strength that I posses. I would never have been able to 'let go' (there is those 2 words again) of pain that I suffered in growing up, and not being able to forgive those who had hurt me. I would never have learned that I have so much to give to life, and to my family, friends, and yes, even strangers. I can smile and say hi to strangers on the street and WOW! I can put a experience has empowered me to become the person that I always wanted to be !

Empowerment is defined as, "to authorize: delegate authority to, to enable; permit." I believe that this is what we have to do to be a survivor. We have to enable and permit ourselves to heal and to open our heart, mind, and soul to our —well-being. Open the door to life and living.

I never asked the question "Why me?" I had always said, "Why not me?" The question for me was why now? I was a newlywed having only been married for fifteen months when I was diagnosed with breast cancer. I believe that there is a reason for everything that happens in our lives, but for the life of me, I could not begin to understand why this was happening to me. Not now! I was not able to fathom a reason until recently.

I have always been a spiritual person, but now I have found that this devastating experience for which there are no answers, has brought me to the point where I know that I have learned to trust in the One who holds all the answers to that haunting questions of why. Just knowing that, is Enough!

Throughout this journey, I was being molded or remolded by someone higher than myself. Throughout the years, there have been pressures or problems, stress or suffering, hurt and heartache, illness or injustice. Now, I felt as if I were being placed in a fire so that the circumstances were heating up with intensity in my life. Suffering has not been wasted. It is not an end in itself. I was hard-pressed on every side, but not crushed or perplexed. I was not in despair, and I felt struck down but not destroyed. As I have reflected on this past year and the story of my loss, it is a manifestation of a universal experience. Loss is a normal part of life, no matter what the loss may be. Experiencing loss is not the defining moment. It is how we respond to that loss that gives meaning to who we are. How we respond will determine the quality, the direction and the impact on our own life and the lives of those all around us.

We recover from different losses as individuals. Recovery does not mean going back to living and how we felt prior to the loss. We learn that we will not live, think, feel or experience things the same way ever again. There is power in response. Response depends upon the choices we make, the grace we receive, and the transformation we experience. It is a life-long journey. Through suffering, our souls become healed.

Being diagnosed with breast cancer has pressed me to the limit. Writing has turned out to be meaningful but has not been the means of my healing. Journaling has. This journey I have been on has only convinced me how long it takes to grow from it. It has reminded me of how meaningful and wonderful life can be. Journaling and reflecting on my thoughts and feelings has resulted in the publication of this book and my previous book. My words may be inadequate, but they have been a reflection. It is a happy result, and not an ending, of this devastating experience. The suffering my family and I have had to endure does not erase the sadness, and the devastation I felt. I don't believe there is anything that can achieve that.

The darkest time for me was not in the beginning of this journey, but came months later. It came when I could not accept my new body image, when I felt lost, out of control, alone, and fearful that I would lose my husband after only fifteen months of marriage. I felt I was in a dingy in a raging, stormy sea being tossed and thrown, unable to understand where I was going, what I was doing, and who I was.

The loss of my breast was catastrophic and its' permanent impact incalculable. Each day has forced me to face some new and devastating dimension of the mastectomy and being diagnosed with breast cancer. It created a whole new context to my life. Even though I am a breast cancer survivor, cancer looms its ominous shadow everyday. It will ebb like the tide, as I have mentioned before, whenever I become ill, or when I have unusual pain or discomfort. I will be reminded every day of what occurred when I look in the mirror and see a different hair color and texture. It looms when my husband touches me and there is no sensation in that breast, or when I notice the different appearance of the breast, and the multiple scars.

There was one day in particular which I believe was my darkest moment. I was ready to give up, stop the chemotherapy, give up on surviving, and just end it all. I was at a point where I had lost my confidence, and my self-esteem. I had no energy to do anything, let alone get dressed. I was in a constant state of despair. I felt I had lost my life and I did not know what was happening or why I was living.

I was taking a walk in the evening. As I walked, the sun was setting. I found myself walking faster, trying to stay in the sunlight, but I was being beaten. There was no way I was going to catch up. Darkness had fallen and it was even darker than I felt. Beaten, I stopped. Standing in the darkness which surrounded me, I was scared. I stood crying. I could not stop crying. I wanted to leave the darkness behind me and find the light, any light, daylight or long-lasting light. I wasn't sure how to find it. It was as if I was in a tunnel without a light at the end. Suddenly, I realized that the fastest way into the light would be going through the darkness. I had no other choice and it was a choice! I could stay in the darkness and let it consume me. I could let it destroy my life or I could walk into it. Through it, I could fight to find my way back .

Walking through the darkness, and allowing myself to grieve, would come to be one of the most difficult things I had to do. The effort would have to be spontaneous and intentional. I would have to share my journey, my sadness, my pain, and my fears. I would also have to make the time to be in solitude with myself everyday and relive what had occurred. I would have to live in the pain and find within it, the grace to survive and eventually grow. The deeper I went into the depth of the pain, I suffered the grief. The more I walked through the darkness, I found that I could live a new life. I could have a different life and in many ways, a better life.

That darkness I felt that I was in, was my own personal loss. I suffered and grieved through it, and tried to find the light. It required that I would have to allow my soul to feel gratitude and joy for the gifts that I *DID* have, and the ability to create a new life. Choice is the key word. I chose to rise above the anguish I felt. I refused to give in to the ultimate power that the stigma of cancer can posses. I wanted to rise above all that, and I wanted to turn my life into an inner triumph.

Many years ago, I remembered reading something in, *Lament for a Son,* by Nicholas Walterstorff, a professor of philosophy. He wrote about his suffering when he lost his son:

> *"And sometimes, when the cry is intense, there emerges a radiance which elsewhere seldom appears: a glow of courage, of love, of insight, of selflessness, of faith. In that radiance we see best what humanity was meant to be...In the valley of suffering, despair and bitterness are brewed. But there also character is made. The valley of suffering is the vale of soul-making"*

I will always suffer and grieve the loss of my breast and live with the fear of the cancer reoccurring. However, what I have learned by walking into the darkness of my grief was that I could appreciate the valuable gifts of life which to me were the love of my husband and children, friendships, working in the yard, weeding the flower beds, and playing the music that I so loved before all this took place. By allowing my soul to grieve and be filled with grace, at the same time, I could resume seeing patients again. I felt the satisfaction and the rewards it had given me in the past. I was able to plant, water and watch nature and all its beauty grow.

When I decided that I would trust God and give up my worries, I began to soar. Soaring is so exhilarating! I became increasingly more willing to leave my comfort zone and live by faith. As I look back at the suffering I have had over the years, I realized that this was no different. At those times, I gave my problems to God and stopped worrying about it. So why should I not do that now? It had made me stronger in my faith, and more consistent in my walk. I drew closer to God and lived more for His glory alone.

As I gave my sorrow and worry to God, He would lift me up to soar above the storms in my life, and even the turmoil that I faced. I started reading the twenty-third Psalm again, as I did many times in my past. This brought me comfort. When I get sad or discouraged, I read the psalm, and I find comfort and peace.

He became involved in every area of my life and showed me miracles I didn't think were possible, such as writing a book and developing a web page for others. I helped others through their difficult time of being diagnosed with breast cancer. I learned how to be a survivor, rather than a victim. I found something that I heard a long time ago and thought about its meaning for me today:

Measure your life by loss and not by gain,
Not by the wine drunk, but by the wine poured forth.
For love's strength standeth in love's sacrifice,
And he who suffers most has the most to give.

We all have different beliefs, but I have learned once again to trust in God! I trust Him when I don't understand. I trust His purpose. I trust Him when my heart is broken. I trust His goodness. I trust Him to know best. I have learned that when I don't understand why, I trust Him because…. God is enough!

What I have found for myself to be true is that God is a universal intelligence, truth and energy that flows between nature and our inner being. If we trust ourselves, we learn how to avoid interfering with nature, other human beings, and even ourselves with our egos.

If we are able to allow this energy to flow in and out of our innermost self, we can bring what we desire to us. If you believe and trust that you are a part of everything, everything will come to you. God is in you as He is in everything around us. All religions have the same beliefs. For example,

- Christianity: The Kingdom of Heaven is within you.

- Islam: Those that know themselves know God.

- Buddhism: Look within, you are Buddha.

- Yoga (part of Hinduism): God dwells within you as you.

To overcome all the obstacles that I have had to face and will continue to face, I pray, knowing God is within me. I ask for strength and inner awareness to be able to handle all that I must and will face. I have to let go of all my fears, my worries and let the Universe take care of itself.

I know my husband is my soul mate because he can push my buttons and get me upset. I am reminded that I am not really in a state of peace. He is my greatest teacher, whether he knows or understands. He is the person I treasure and I thank God for sending him into my life! I know this sounds rather strange, but because he can send me into turmoil, it only shows me I still have a lot of work to do. I will have to keep working to allow my inner self, and the universal energy to flow within me.

What I have also come to realize is that it has given me a purpose again. When I was a case manager, my purpose was to make my patients comfortable, provide support, guidance and education so that they would be able to move through the end-of-life process. I helped the family members cope with the dying process. When I became a team supervisor, I was no longer connected to patients and families, and I lost my purpose. I lost the personal satisfaction of sharing love and hope. I lost my sense of pride because I was not directly involved with making life better for others.

While home for those many months, and even when returning to work, I felt that I was insignificant. I felt like I had failed. I was afraid that I would not be able to continue in hospice. I was lost. I knew I had to find another means to pull myself out of the rut I had found myself in.

As nurses, we are the mothering, nurturing type personalities, and we want to make everything better. I needed to be able to touch other lives, to make a difference in someone's life. I needed to "reach out and touch someone," as the saying goes. I wanted to give someone else's life story a happy ending, and give them hope.

I think each person is part of a giant jigsaw puzzle, and we don't know the value of our own little piece until something devastating happens to us. We probably carry a piece of someone else's puzzle as well. To release the burden that I was shouldering, I needed to invest my life and give significance to the breast cancer. Only then would I be able to make a difference in someone else's life.

Mother Teresa said, "Few of us can do great things, but all of us can do small things with great love." Sharing my journey with those who read my story is my small, but significant gift to help others find hope. I was not being punished. I was given an opportunity to realize my strength and ability to continue, to help others, and to share goodness and love. I was spending too much time worrying about something that I could not change. I chose to have a mastectomy and chemotherapy, because I wanted to continue to live. So instead of the cancer becoming a death sentence, closing the door to life, I allowed it to open the door. I decided to empower the cancer in a positive direction! This did not happen right away.

It took months and a lot of soul-searching before I could take control of my life and not let the cancer control me. When I decided to be in control, I was less fearful and I was more spontaneous. I was not so judgmental of myself and others, and my ability not to worry was fading. I started smiling from the heart because I was more connected to myself, my mind, and others. I could extend the love in my heart outside my family and let others love me in return. Now I just let things happen and do not try to make them happen.

The diagnosis of breast cancer with all the emotions, feelings and fears gave light to the significance and purpose of my life. It gave me the gift of hope and love to those who have begun this journey or are about to go through it. It helps them find inner peace. It is to help those with friends who have breast cancer to understand what they fear, the emotional rollercoaster they are on, and to let them know that once all the surgeries and treatments are over, that is when they need their friends. It is then that we have time to think about what really happened and how it has affected our lives and life.

My writing has become my way of learning more of who I am. Where it takes me is thrilling because I learn something from the expressions on paper that are deep within my heart and soul. Writing has become a means of healing for me, and I hope that these written words will help you and others know that we can celebrate life after breast cancer. It takes time, patience, and understanding to learn that breast cancer does not have to be the end of life. It can be the beginning!

Writing allows me to share this journey with those who have and have not been down this path. It helps others understand what it is that we feel and think. It informs those who take care of the dying and their families, gives guidelines for what is needed for support, and helps to remind friends and family members that after the treatment is over is when we need them the most.

After I found the article, "The Best Day Of My Life," I read it every day. In fact, I have hung it up on the bathroom mirror! It gives me the ability to take on a different thought process—positive thinking and soul rejuvenation. I started feeling better about myself and what had happened to me. I started to use this experience as a means, and a catalyst, to find new meaning, and a new life. It brought a sense of purpose and I was less afraid as the days turned into weeks and months.

A dear friend sent the following message to me over the Internet, and it is priceless. It is entitled,

100-yard dash

Some people understand life better.
And they call some of these people "retarded"…

At the Seattle Special Olympics, nine contestants,
All physically or mentally disabled, assembled at the
Starting line for the 100-yard dash.

At the gun, they all started out, not exactly in a dash,
But with a relish to run the race to the finish and win.
All that is, except one little boy who stumbled on the asphalt,
Tumbled over a couple of times, and began to cry.

The other eight heard the boy cry.
They slowed down and looked back.
Then they all turned around and went back....
Every one of them!

One girl with Down's Syndrome bent down and kissed him and said,
"This will make it better."
Then all nine linked arms and walked together to the finish line.

Everyone in the stadium stood. The cheering went on for
Several minutes.
People who were there are still telling the story...
Why? Because deep down we know this one thing:

What matters in this life is more than winning ourselves.
What matters in this life is helping others win, even if it
Means slowing down and changing our course.
A candle loses nothing by lighting another candle!

I thought about what this was saying to me and I realized that once again, cancer had been a gift! It has slowed me down, changed my course in life, and made me realize that I had something to offer—to help others fight to be a survivor. It made me realize what I was missing living my present life. I needed to get in touch with my inner self, that spiritual self. I needed to connect my body and mind, and find the peace that I really had been searching for. I want to make sure that those who have been diagnosed, or soon to be diagnosed with breast cancer, that they know that they are not alone. There are thousands of us out there, who have learned to cope in different ways, and fought the fight to be a survivor.

I have started giving more thought about going back to the field as a case manager. I want to work with patients and their families through the end-of-life process. I want to help them find peace and help them cope with the loss of their loved one. I believe that is my gift to offer others. It's not about managing a team of nurses, but rather, it's about being out there with them, supporting patients and families.

I am fascinated with the teachings of the Dalai Lama. The following is what he said for 2005. Think deeply after reading each step, and I believe that you will see a path that will lead to a new strength as I have found.

Instructions for Life

1. Take into account that great love and great achievements, involve great risks.
2. When you lose, don't lose the lesson.
3. Follow the Three R's:
    > Respect for self
    > Respect for others and
    > Responsibility for all your actions
4. Remember that not getting what you want is sometimes a wonderful stroke of luck.
5. Learn the rules so you know how to break them properly.
6. Don't let a little dispute injure a great relationship.
7. When you realize you've made a mistake take immediate steps to correct it.
8. Spend some alone time every day.
9. Open arms to change, but don't let go of your values.
10. Remember that silence is sometimes the best answer.
11. Live a good, honorable life, then when you get older and think back, you'll be able to enjoy it a second time.
12. A loving atmosphere in your home is the foundation of your life.
13. In disagreements with loved ones, deal only with the current situation. Don't bring up the past.
14. Share your knowledge. It's a way to achieve immortality.
15. Be gentle with the Earth.
16. Once a year, go someplace you've never been before.
17. Remember that the best relationship is one in which your love for each

other exceeds your need for each other.
18. Judge your success by what you had to give up in order to get it.
19. Approach love and cooking with reckless abandon.

Buddhist beliefs are very simple, as is Christianity. It is all based on love and kindness to all things around us. It is very much like the American Indians. They believe that all life and energy comes from "Mother Earth" and we are immortal. Our bodies are just a vessel for our soul and spirit. When our body dies, our spirit is still alive. The voice of the Native American Indian in the following prayer is uplifting. It teaches us that our lessons are to be learned in the power and the energy of nature. If we listen to the wind and behold the beauty of creation, then we realize that we are of the same beauty as individuals. We are in this prayer. We need to reflect on the energy, the spirit of our surroundings and use its positive energy to give us strength and courage, and to give us comfort. Our greatest enemy is our self!

O Great Spirit, Hear Us

O Great Spirit whose voice we hear in the winds
And whose breath gives us life
to all the world.
Hear Us. We are small and weak.
We come with you in mind to find strength and
wisdom.
Let us walk in beauty
And make our eyes
Ever behold the sunset.
Make our hands respect
The things you have made,
And our ears sharp to hear your voice.
Make us wise
So that we may understand
The things you have taught our relatives.
Let us learn the lessons you have hidden in every
leaf and rock.
We seek strength,
Not to be greater than our brothers and sisters,
But to fight our greatest enemy - ourselves.
Make us always ready to come to you
With clean hands and straight eyes.
So when life fades, as the fading sunset, our spirit
may come to you
Without shame.

-Native American Prayer

I really believe that if we live our lives as if there is no tomorrow, we will know how to pass from this life to another. We will show our family and friends that we will live on through them. We will have passed on knowledge and a strength that was ours, and now theirs to live their life joyously—to dance if no one is watching.

I spoke of having a web site earlier, and how it came to be. It is called the Celebration of Life. It is dedicated and designed to bring resources and information to anyone who has been diagnosed with breast cancer, or those who have a family member or friend with breast cancer. It allows anyone who has fears, questions and concerns to ask questions and know that there is someone on the other end who knows exactly how they feel. I have been there and will know where their emotions are taking them. It is a place to share your journey.

I am by no means a licensed counselor, but a counselor through experience. I have learned how to be a survivor, and have found strength I never knew I had. It has been a healing process for me and I want to be able to help others with what I have learned. If I am able to only help one person, then I have achieved my purpose. Reaching out to others in a time of need, giving support, validating someone's feelings, and helping them reach inner peace is a driving force within me. It is the sense of urgency I had less than a year ago.

Having breast cancer did not close the door to life! It opened a new door full of wonder, and allowed me to find inner peace that I have never known before. It has given me strength and the determination to fight and survive. With a new sense of purpose, I realize that life is too short to worry about those things that I cannot control. It is far more important to help others, giving the love that we have within us to those who need a smile, a hug, or a kind word and gesture.

I have taken a risk that I probably would never have done, and that was to write a book about my journey. I wanted to share it with others so that I could find my way back to a new normal, and give the love and compassion to those who have started down this path, as well as to those who are in the midst of it.

Chapter Seven

Drawn By The Gentle Pull Of My Heart

Whenever two ways lie before
Us, one of which is easy and the
Other hard, one of which requires
No exertion while the other calls
For resolution and endurance,
Happy are those who choose the
Mountain path and scorn the
Thought of resting in the valley.
These are the men and women
Who are destined in the end to
Conquer and succeed.
-Author Unknown

I decided to take on a healthy attitude. I needed to be definite in what I wanted in terms of health care. I had made the decision to change oncologists because there was no connection between us and I was not getting my questions answered. I decided to have genetic counseling and testing so that I would know the best type of follow-up for me.

I changed the way that I ate. I stopped eating red meat and now eat only fresh vegetables, fish and poultry. I only buy organic foods. I do not want to introduce pesticides into my body. I eat smaller portions and only eat until I am comfortable. I have started walking at least three times a week and sometimes more. As I walk, I take in the beauty of my surroundings, and fill my mind with pleasant thoughts. This helps me rid myself of unwanted feelings of sadness and fear. It has given me new energy. I consume at least two liters of water a day, which keeps me hydrated. It flushes out all the "poisons" as I call it, and it really does make me feel better.

The chemotherapy had caused some toenails to die. I cut them short and as they started re-growing, I decided that I would do something that I have never done before. I got a pedicure. Wow! What a relaxing experience to sit in the chair with your feet in warm water and then have your feet and legs massaged. As I sat there, I decided I was going to have that done at least twice a month. It was something that I would do for me, treating myself to one of those little pleasures of life.

I know that I am loved by a multitude of people. To love others, I had to learn how to love the new me, and I could only do that by finding inner peace. I had to take control of my life and my destiny. This disease was not a death sentence, but my door to a new life!

I explained this in my previous book that every day I would stand in front of the mirror and find something positive to say about how I looked. I started with my hair. I found that it took several days to say that it looked all right, and then I was able to go to work and be in public without a wig.

The difficulty came when I stood there looking at my breasts. They were so different looking and it made me cry. However, I would not leave that position until I found three things that I liked. I still have to look in the mirror and appreciate what they look like. It doesn't mean that I still don't miss my old breasts and wish that I had them back. At least I am able to say that I look all right.

Wearing a bra, I found that no one could tell what had happened to me. Surprisingly to me, after a year, I felt that my breasts were now a part of me. They were no longer something unfamiliar and strange. My hair grew back, and most people would think that it was just cut very short. It is a different texture, color and thickness, but it is something that only I know that is different.

Many people marvel at how quickly it is growing. In the beginning, I would respond that it was not growing fast enough. Now I find myself excited and saying, "Yeah!" By Christmas, it should be five inches long! What is even more exciting is to realize that your thought process is changing. You are more accepting of the new body image. That is exciting because you are healing and getting through the grief.

I have a dimple for a belly button but having a real-looking belly button was of least importance. A belly button is just a scar and that is what I have, a dimpled scar. No one knows or can see that.

Getting dressed for work, I stand in the mirror and find three things every morning that are positive about the way that I look when dressed. Looking attractive again seemed to play an important part in how I felt about going to work. I started wearing make-up because I was pale. I thought that without make-up, I looked ill. I didn't want people to think that I was sick. It also helped remove the fatigue look that I have. However, by the end of my workday, everyone knew that I was tired.

I bought new clothing for work for two reasons. The old ones did not fit any longer, and I needed to have things which didn't remind me of how I looked before the mastectomy. My head would play games with me when I wore the clothing that I had before. My heart would sink and I would feel empty and sad. Buying new clothes was my way of controlling what this disease had done to me.

In the evening, when I took my shower and dressed, I would stand there and find three things that were positive about how I looked in my nightwear. There was no difference than before the surgery. It was just in my head that I looked different. Neither my husband nor myself could see the scars or the breasts under my clothing. This process took several months, and I still have days that I do not feel comfortable with the way that I look. Those days are fewer and far between now.

Dr. Anne Borik has written a wonderful book, *Sign Chi Do*. It is an exercise created and designed by her to harmonize the universal language of sign with movement. It allows you to attain true relaxation, and helps you connect your mind and spirit so that you have a sense of total well-being. There is an exciting movement of energy when practiced between the body and mind when they are in harmony with one another.

This exercise that she demonstrates in her book helped me concentrate on good health and allows me to give up my anxiety and depression. It allows me to convey love to everyone, and to accept love and find peace within myself. It rebuilt my confidence and I was motivated to proclaim my freedom to survive breast cancer. Once I found inner peace, I could find a new sense of independence and willingness to take on life. I was going to control my life, not the cancer.

What I discovered was that I was already a survivor. However, survivorship needs to be nurtured. Hearing we are going to be all right, and that we are going to be cancer-free soon, helps our belief system. We are sure we are going to beat the odds. We are going to win! This thought is contagious. I reminded myself everyday that I was going to win. I would survive! I thanked God for allowing me to live and enjoy the life that He had given to me.

My heart filled with love for others. I learned that loving is not just for family. It is for friends, neighbors and others, such as Dr. Geoffrey, whom I adore very much. He has been a major source of my lifeline and I am very grateful to him for his compassion, kindness and caring attitude that he showed to me. A whole new world opened up to me when I began to love myself, because it allowed others to love me. I now had more support than I ever dreamed possible.

I refused to perceive the diagnosis of breast cancer as a death sentence. I made it a personal responsibility to take care of my health. I did research on breast cancer to find what I could do to take better care of myself. I learned how I should eat and exercise, and I learned how to stay relaxed. The diagnosis of breast cancer gave me a commitment to live. It gave me a purpose. The mind has great power over the body. I used breast cancer as a catalyst to find new meaning and purpose to my life. This has taken me on a path of healing and love and has taught others how to live.

To help me survive, I read a book about Aide's patients. In it, Max Navarre, one of the contributing editors of Surviving and Thriving with Aides, said, "If you have never loved yourself, never really loved yourself, gently and unconditionally, now is the time to do that. Love yourself, forgive yourself, and at the same time, know there is nothing to forgive." What I realized was that I wasn't being punished with this dreadful disease for something that I had done. I had done nothing. It just happened!

I had to love myself unconditionally, and find others who loved me the same. Unconditional love is a real safety net. I thought about my children when they were little. I told them that I may be angry with them, but I loved them no matter what they did. My love for them was unconditional. The same holds true for ourselves. We have to love ourselves unconditionally and then amazing things happen. When we feel safe and secure, wonderful things can be done. Miracles do happen every day!

Life does not owe us anything, but we can give of our talents and energy. We can share our heart-felt emotions. We can embrace intimacy and sexuality as an expression of who we are. Life is our Gift, and we need to share that and ourselves with others. Only then will we see the extraordinary in the ordinary. Only then will we be able to turn a negative experience into one that is positive. We have to learn from mistakes, bad choices, from our fears, and from life-threatening diseases.

When my husband leaves for work at five in the morning, I now go for a walk. When I get home, I get in the hot tub and relax. I use the trigger word that I was given to take me to my safe place to find peace. I then get ready for work. I really don't want to work anymore, but we are not in a financial position which would allow me to retire from nursing.

The vegetarian diet is not bad. In fact, it is pretty good. I do not feel full, just comfortable, and I am starting to lose weight. I have gained so much weight since the chemotherapy, that it is time that I start to get it off once again. I walk four to five blocks, three times a week. I think that the diet and exercise are starting to make me feel better physically. My muscles hurt less, and when I walk, there is an increase in the endurance that I didn't have before. The medication that was prescribed has been helping also. While I walk, I listen to myself breathe. I empty my head of thought and feel myself relax. I listen to the birds, rustling of the leaves in the breeze. I enjoy the sight of the cactus and flowering plants. I enjoy the smell of grills cooking food, watch the sunset and know that these ordinary sights are extraordinary.

Chapter Eight

Going Beyond Into The Impossible
Finding New Strength Through My Pain

At the onset of this journey, I focused on the physical aspect of what breast cancer meant. I became aware when I was coming to the end of that first year. Physically I was healed but my inner self was still in turmoil. I still felt lost because I did not know who I was, and where I was going with my time left on this earth.

I had been denying the emotional pain that I felt losing my breast, and being diagnosed with breast cancer. I tried to manage our home and do normal activities. Eventually, this denial of pain finally won. I was no longer able to deny the pain. It was unbearable. I had journaled and when reading it over repeatedly, I found I had gone through nearly every stage of grief—not once, but several times. I believe that I will continue to grieve for years to come. I will be reminded every day of the loss of my breast when I dress and undress, when I look in the mirror and see a reflection of someone with a different hair color and texture, and when I pick up the bottle of anti-estrogen medication.

I fell deep into what felt like a black whole of emptiness, and I was still felt the dread and despair. I was constantly crying and unable to sleep. I was afraid to have my husband see me without hair and to have him touch me. I was afraid to meet new people, and to face my co-workers. I was in such a deep, dark hole that I was even afraid to have my family home for Christmas.

Depression, a treatable disease, came from denying my pain and my anger. I denied my soul to feel pain and joy at the same time. I denied my soul to grow. When I made the choice, and as I have previously stated, choice is the keyword, I chose to walk through the darkness, face my mortality, and allowed my soul to feel pain and joy simultaneously. When I was able to *stop* being a nurse, I could return to the light. I was able to feel happiness and joy, along with the sadness and despair.

I eventually found that pain to be a gift. Whether we feel pain from the loss of a loved one, or the loss of a breast, or even other body parts I would think would apply. The pain can be unbearable at times. Pain is a gift because it shows us we are able to feel, whether the pain is physical or in our souls. Pain of loss is severe because it shows us the pleasure life gives to us, or the value of what was lost.

Then something jumped out at me when I looked at the word 'cancer.' It begins with the word...can! It was then that I realized that I needed to find my inner spiritual self to heal. I believe that I was partly there when I was diagnosed with breast cancer and knew that it was not an end to life, but a path to a new beginning. I can never answer the question, "Why now?" I have to believe and trust there was a lesson to learn. I believe that it was to lead me on this path of finding my inner spiritual self.

When life as we know it comes crashing down on us, our hearts ache for ourselves, and our family. We seem to go numb to the things going on around us. I think I was even in shock. My faith had been tested, and sometimes when I was going through chemotherapy, I didn't know if I could go on. I knew, however, that I had to and I knew that I could!

I thought of ways that would help me heal. As I have written this book and *Surviving Breast Cancer*, I awoke to those things that I had done to help me heal. I learned to accept my feelings and know that it was all right to feel the way that I did. I didn't push them out of my mind. I spent quiet time alone, and wrote in my journal. I described what I was feeling and why, and then I would cry or just reflect on those feelings.

I would talk about what I was feeling to Diana and LouAnne, and they would reaffirm what I was feeling. Then they would guide me to find some peace and comfort. I had to share my pain and my journey because only then would I be able to know that I was not alone.

I mentioned in my first book that I stopped people from telling me sad stories. To this day, I still cannot listen to really sad stories. I do make new memories, write poems and give them to people that I really care about. I write letters to people to let them know how much I appreciate them.

I have always had a special love for angels, and I started really collecting angels and books. They are all over the house, and in the yard. When I glance at one of them, I say a prayer of thanks that I am still here to enjoy life, and to thank them for their guidance and protection.

I am now a "hugger!" I have shared someone else's grief with them, held them when they were hurting and crying. I started to enjoy the little things. I think that the two most important things that I learned was that I had to live each day one day at a time and in ways that were meaningful. I had to take the time to allow myself to heal, and to take the time to feel and learn to do things for myself. Immanuel Kant said it best, "The greatest human quest is to know what one must do in order to become a human being." I was not allowing myself to feel human. I felt mutilated and deformed. I only looked at the outside of myself and not the inside.

My emotions were on a roller coaster that I could not seem to control. I wrote my first book, *Surviving Breast Cancer*, as a means to heal and to share my journey with others in hopes of touching someone's life. I did not write it to make money. It was to give of myself to help others. It allowed me to find ways to become at peace with myself. In some ways, it did not accomplish what I thought that it would. I still felt an urgency that I could not understand. There was an energy that I was missing. That energy and urgency was to find who I am, to free myself of the wasted energy of worry, and to be able to accept myself as who I am right now.

In each moment, we are free to decide. I needed to decide that I could look inside myself and find that energy I was sensing or missing. I believe what I am trying to describe is an inner force, spiritual or enlightenment. I had been on a physical journey that not only affected my outer self, but the inner self. I relied on my intelligence as a nurse to be my guide, and found that was not helpful. In fact, it was probably more harmful. I had to learn to love, forgive, and to be kind to myself so those qualities would radiate outward and overflow to others. What I found was that I needed to know who I am, what I am doing here in this body, and at this point in my life.

I was afraid of failing. I came to learn that I couldn't fail at anything because everything I do will produce a result. Labeling myself as a failure was wasted energy. It was meaningless and it was a negative attitude. I was afraid to suffer and of becoming the cause of my family's suffering. However, with suffering comes hope, joy, and new memories.

Sitting Bull described the power of love in the following words, "Behold, my brother, the spring has come; the Earth has received the embraces of the sun. And we shall soon see the results of that I love! Every seed is awakened and so has all the animal life! It is through this mysterious power that we too have our being."

These words helped me become the person I was looking for in the mirror's reflection. The fear, the doubt, frustration and sadness of the person I could no longer see, because my life was taking on new form. I was able to see and feel hope and joy. Inner contentment was coming into full swing with whom I was transforming into.

I allowed myself to bring my feelings to the surface. I talked to those fears and doubts as if they were a person. It allowed me to dominate them because I had renewed strength, courage and love within myself. They would just walk away, so to speak. So when they start to creep back into my mind, I let them come forward to the surface. I hold onto my new belief and they fade away.

As I consider the emotional spiritual being that I have become, I am reminded that I may not have lost who I was. I have just transcended to another level. My body, although in the process of natural and surgical changes, is a vessel for my heart and soul. When I separate the body from the mind, my body continues to function. It is as if I am standing outside myself as an observer.

I learned to become aware of that part of me that's invisible to the eye. Who I am is not the body that I carry around that is always changing and shifting. It is the inner self that never changes and is hidden in a changing world. Becoming self-aware is discovering one's higher self, and being able to live joyously, giving yourself peace and fulfillment.

Dr. Andrew Weil, in his book, *Self Healing,* recommends positive imagery. If you really think about it, worry is the most common form. After reading some of his work, I decided that I would replace that negative imagery with positive ones. I would only allow myself a few moments a day to worry. I would write them down. Each week, I would go back and read what I had written. I found that many of those fears never came to pass.

Dr. Weil also suggests that to help with healing, whether physical or emotional, that you visualize yourself healing. I practiced this, spending thirty minutes everyday just sitting, with my eyes closed, and meditating. I would relax every muscle in my body, starting at my head and going down slowly until I eventually reached my toes. You must breathe slowly and deeply, letting all the air out. I would ask the angels of healing to come at that moment and remove everything that did not belong in my body. I would ask them to remove the anxiety and confusion and allow me to heal. Belleruth Naparstek's, *A Meditation to Promote a Successful Surgery,* also discusses how to use positive imagery. You can visit healthjourenys.com to obtain more information.

Self- hypnosis is also very effective. When I enter my 'safe place' that is what I am doing. I am putting myself in a trance-like state, which reduces the anxiety that I feel. It allows me to feel better physically and emotionally. I feel that I am worthy of life, living and love. I know that I am healing.

This self-hypnosis can also be used before surgery. It has been shown that it can reduce surgical pain, anxiety, nausea and vomiting, and decreases the duration of the hospital stay. Dr. Steven Gurevich's, *Surgery and Recovery,* discusses this process and how it can help to reduce the amount of pain and complications following surgery. It has been proven that it can reduce the development of blood clots in patients, and it reduces the amount of blood loss during surgery. Please visit transformation.com for more information. A book that would be helpful if you are having surgery, is by Peggy Huddleston, *Prepare for Surgery, Heal Faster* (Angel River Press, 2002).

There are two other techniques that can be used, although more studies need to be done. Many people, including myself, find that energy techniques such as Therapeutic Touch and Reiki help them heal faster after surgery. These therapies, which involve no touching or light touching to balance a person's energy field, are certainly relaxing. They may boost immunity and relieve pain.

Many nurses now practice therapeutic touch in hospitals. I was seeing a massage therapist for fibromyalgia and she would use these methods. Brushing is a technique, which involves only light touching and it is as if you are brushing the limbs of the body ever so lightly. My legs would hurt so bad, but when she would do this, the pain would dissipate.

For a month prior to one of the surgeries that I had to have, she did Reiki on the abdominal scar from the original surgery. Without being touched, there was a warm flow of energy that emanated from my abdomen. It broke up the adhesions that were just below the scar. The week before surgery, I felt the scar and I could barely feel the adhesions that had been there. The new suture line healed without any problems.

I remember saying that everything happens for a reason. There are no accidents or coincidences. Everything that shows up in our lives has a purpose, and a lesson to be learned. Learning to control the fear was difficult. Even if I did not understand it, I had to learn to let it go. Only then would I find peace and contentment.

I started to see the extraordinary in the ordinary. I am in awe when I go out in evening and look up at the stars, seeing the moon and the light with which it radiates. I like getting up early in the morning to watch the sunrise and listen to the birds' cheery songs. I thank God for the best day of my life!

Sitting in silence is probably the best gift that we can give ourselves. We become one with the world around us. Herman Melville wrote, *"Silence is the only Voice of our God…. All profound things and emotions of things are preceded and attended by Silence."* By sitting in silence, and shifting away from the noise that surrounds me, I could find the answers that I was searching for and the guidance that I needed.

Meditation was difficult in the beginning, but I made a place in our garden for meditation. I try to go there daily to focus on my inner self, and to obtain peace and contentment. I try to let go of my fears that consume me, and let the energy of life fill my soul. I told you previously that I have used flower visualization to help me relax. I thought of another visualization that I had remembered seeing, and I realized that I needed to try it because it was of angels. I believe and trust in my angels that surround me. So I knew that I needed to really get in touch with them and allow their peace and energy to fill my soul.

To try this meditation, I suggest that you play some very soft mood relaxation music. An example would be the sounds of water. It doesn't matter what type of relaxation sound you use, as long as when you close your eyes and listen to the music, that it takes you away to a safe place. You should feel your body molding into the chair in which you sit.

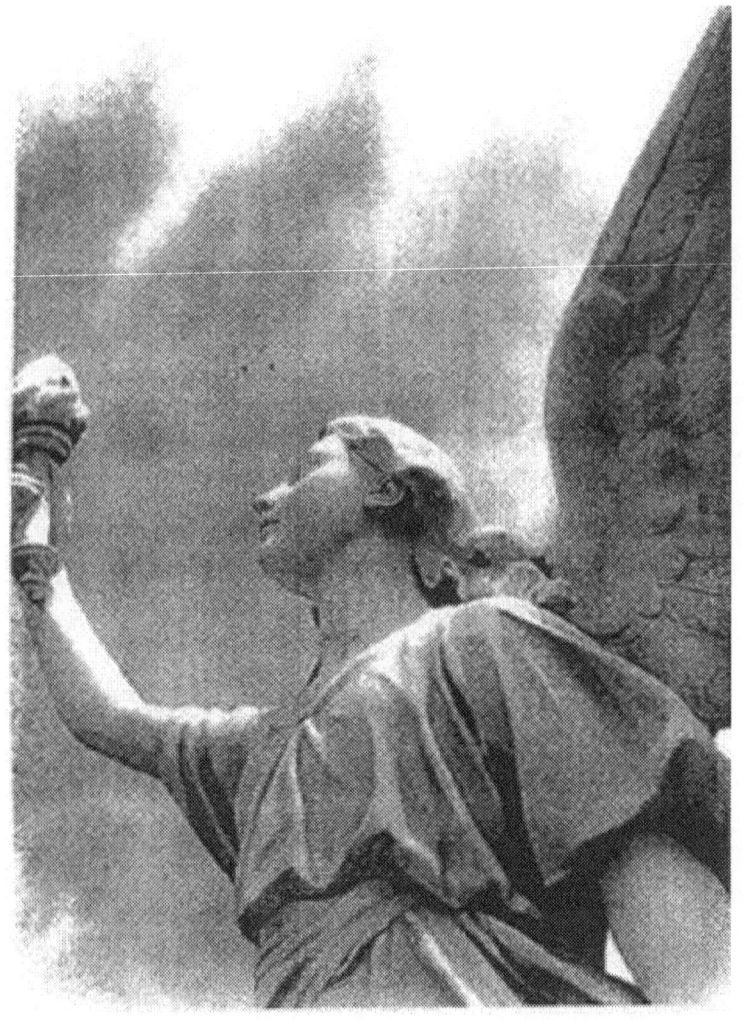

Angel Visualization

Imagine yourself with wings,
soaring high above the clouds.
You are weightless and completely
free. You are filled with energy
and excitement. The feeling is
exhilarating!

When you are relaxed and
confident, your body will become
light, rising higher and higher.
If you become tense and fearful,
your body will become heavy,
sinking lower and lower.

Allow yourself to soar freely
with your arms outstretched.
Feel the wind in your hair, the
sun on your face. You feel
completely liberated!

I like this visualization because it connects me with my guardian angels and the energy of the Universe. When I am soaring high in the clouds, I feel so light and liberated. It is as if there in nothing that can touch me. I can feel the energy flowing in and out of me. When I return, I feel like I was Wendy from Peter Pan, soaring higher and higher. I can take myself to my safe place, create new things to appear that help me relax and give pleasure to my senses of touch, smell, and visual.

I am sure that some of you who read this will think or believe that I have lost my mind. Or, you might think that I need to be put in a white straight jacket and taken to an asylum. But before you do that, try it. Practice it when you are afraid, when you feel lost, and when you are sad and alone. This exercise puts you in touch with your very own soul.

Souls are not the spiritual part of us that exists only at death. It is an ever-present part of us that guides our being, and which allows us to connect and feel the energy of the Universe. It is the source for healing our emotional pain that we have had to endure. It teaches us who we are. It allows us to hope and dream the impossible. Our soul not only allows us, it teaches us to love ourselves and to offer that love to others in the simplest of forms. When we offer to help anyone, even for a moment, we allow ourselves to extend our love that exists in our souls, to someone who is in need.

It is strange to speak of myself in the past tense, but the person that I was, is a friend that has now passed through my life. I treasure that person, but I have found a new friend, the new me! She finds that there are more "little pleasures" in life than she expected to find. She is able to enjoy every moment, and is able to be more peaceful and content with the way things are right now, today!

Finding the inner beauty that I have within myself was difficult, and it took a long time. Now, though, I am able to allow others to see it. I am able to share it. It radiates in my smile, my hugs, and in what I give of myself to others without asking for something in return.

I had to stop judging myself for my appearance now. I had to learn to be myself. Whatever I was in the past, whatever behaviors, whether good or bad that had occurred, there was a lesson in them. I mentioned previously that I had gotten rid of the backpack that I was carrying. It contained all the bad experiences I have had, and all the guilt. I sat and thought about them and realized that there was a lesson in all of them and I had learned from them. I was getting rid of my history.

I now feel that these new breasts are part of me and not something that is foreign. I can look at myself and I know that I am a whole person, and having a reconstructed breast only changed in appearance to me. How I look on the outside in clothing has not changed. In fact, when I think about it, I look even better because I now have a waist and no belly! I lost all that saggy skin and fat with the "tummy tuck" that was done to make the breast. I laugh at myself because I always wanted to get rid of that apron from having babies, but I never did anything about it. Wow! What an adventure to lose all that is how I look at it! Now, it is a loss that I have made a memorial to, I suppose.

I have an inner desire to meet the needs of others rather than those of myself. I am learning how to be me. I think Albert Schweitzer said it best, *"Every man has to seek in his own way to make his own self more noble and to realize his own true worth. You must give some time to your fellow man. Even if it's a little thing, do something for those who have need of help, something for which you get no pay but the privilege of doing it. For remember, you don't live in a world all your own. Your brothers are here, too."* I am learning that life has unlimited possibilities! Florinda Donner's definition of freedom in her book, *Being-In-Dreaming*, states that *"Freedom will cost you the mask you have on. The mask that feels so comfortable and is so hard to shed off, not because it fits so well but because you have been wearing it for so long. Freedom is the total absence of concern about yourself."*

Once I stopped worrying about myself and began concentrating on helping others, I found the inner peace that I was searching for. My husband always says that there is no one as free, and one who has nothing to lose. He is right. If I am free, then I have the ability and the inner resources to be at peace with who I am right now. I had to take the time to appreciate all the beauty in this world, and in others. I could not be judgmental any longer. I had to let go of the conflict within myself and stop asking, "Why now?"

As I sit in my little area of meditation, I have to look at all the emotions that were part of a problem that I carried—fear, sadness, anger, and pain. Then I had to decide that I didn't want those emotions. They were controlling me. I had to take control and decide that they were unwanted. It was those feelings that put me in the emotional roller coaster that I was on. As I let go of those emotions, not seeing them as bad or good, and using them as energy, I was able to find a solution to the problem.

I have started walking in the early morning and then again in the evening. I look at everything and see beauty in things that I never saw before. I breathe deeply and marvel at the foothills because I have never seen them so green. I have never seen the desert so beautiful! I listen to the birds sing as I walk and I start to feel my steps becoming light, as if I were starting to walk in the air. It is like I am becoming one with nature, and one with myself. I am not sure. Maybe I have just found my spiritual self.

As a breast cancer survivor, I know nothing will ever be the same. I will always have sadness with my loss. There will always be the "cancer worry," but I will not be afraid to share my journey. At the end of that dark tunnel was light. The light was a new light of strength, a new happiness, a new awareness of who I am, and who I was becoming.

I have learned to trust God completely and I understand that God's energy is within and around me. Each moment and each day is a gift. Cancer, and all the emotional pain, has been a gift. It has opened a new life, and a new beginning so I can see the extraordinary in the ordinary. It has been in the valley of darkness that I have found inner strength that I did not know that I had. I found courage to go on with my life and I'm learning how to live again!

Another Chance

There is never a dull moment
When God wakes me every morn
For it's time to start a new day
It's time to weather any storm

I consider it a countless blessing
When awaking to each a new day
And each breathe that I am given
A chance to change, what I do or say

Another chance I have been given
To help the hungry, and the lost
To help another should realize
They were loved, and paid form with a cost

No, there is never a dull moment
When God wakes every morn
For this new day will be better
Thank the one before

Debbie Looney
10-06-2005

I would like to thank Debbie Looney for her inspirational writing of "Another Chance" who willingly allowed me to use her beautiful work to appear in my book. She writes inspirational poetry on the web to help others, and touch hearts with her God given talent. Debbie resides in Michigan with her Husband Doug, and is the mother of 4 grown children, and a grandmother to 13 wonderful Grandchildren.

Chapter Nine

The Universe Will Work In Unison With You

Prayer for Protection

The Light of God surrounds me;
The Love of God enfolds me;
The Power of God protects me;
The Presence of God watches over me;
Wherever I am, God is,
And all is well.
-James Dillet Freeman

When I was working for hospice, we had a male certified nursing assistant. His name was Steve. He was always in my office telling me how his day went, and the problems he had. He was a good soul. He was very kind and compassionate. He would invite patients who did not have family in town to holiday meals, and he would buy patients and families food and paper products if they were in financial need.

It was some time after I had been back to work when I learned that he was an ordained minister. He never asked how I was feeling or doing but would ask one of my co-workers if I was all right and if I appeared to be having a bad week. Occasionally, he would bring me apple cobbler that he had not eaten for lunch.

It was a few weeks after I had resigned that he called me in the evening at home. He wanted our street address. He said that he wanted to send me something. We talked for awhile about his family and himself, and how things were going at work. He had been ill for a few weeks and we spoke about that. He was very sad that I had left. He wanted to send me something that he had given to people in the past, and that had been very comforting to them. He thought I would enjoy it. Without hesitation, I gave him our address.

In a couple of days, I received a package from a Christian bookstore. It was a book, *I Am With You Always,* by Chip Ingram. I skimmed through the book and came upon a chapter that really made some sense to me. My thoughts and behaviors were an escape from reality and they made me feel guilty for what had happened. I felt guilty because I thought I had let my husband down, and that I had disappointed him. It was as if I asked for this disease or that I was being punished for something that I had done in my past—a wrong behavior, a wrong choice, bad language or thoughts. I had stopped remembering all the blessings that I had been given throughout my life.

When we are down, right down on the floor, so depressed that we feel we are alone and there is no hope, we are thinking negatively, and we are actually thinking about ourselves. It is insidious and ugly when we have put all our attention on ourselves. We become ungrateful in our upward focus, negative in our inward focus, and insensitive in our outward focus toward others. I had to lift my soul and take a positive step so that I could be positive with others.

I sat down to think about all my blessings that I have had in my life. I looked at photo albums, wedding pictures, some really good pictures of my sons and why that moment in time was so special to me. I reminisced about the vacations that we had taken. I read my journal, and thought about all those whom I love. I thought about the special people who have come and gone in my life, and the gifts they brought to me when I was in need.

The truth is, 'Today is not the worst day in my life, or yours!' I had the choice to redirect my thoughts, rather than give in to my feelings. I was letting fear rule. The dictionary defines fear as a sudden attack, anxiety, or agitation caused by the presence of danger, evil, or pain. It covers a wide range of emotions, such as timidity, apprehension, terror, or dread. Most of us don't need a dictionary to tell us what fear is. We all have had fear in our lives. The word "cancer" puts fear in our hearts and mind at the moment it is spoken. It will turn our world upside down without notice. We fear the loss of a body part, illness, pain, dying, death or the dying or death of a loved one. I thought about all the fears that breast cancer brought, such as disfigurement, loss of my husband, loss of my hair, fear of fatigue and illness, and pain. I feared dying only in the sense that I didn't want to leave those whom I loved—my new husband and my sons.

I had to turn myself around! I was the one who feared intimacy. I was the one who felt disfigured. It was me who felt I could no longer contribute to my marriage and was unattractive to my husband. I was not going to allow myself to be a victim of a disease, allowing it to take me to a living grave. I was going to forge through the darkness to the light and be victorious! I was going to be a survivor! I was not going to allow cancer to destroy my sense of hope.

The fight had started. I was going to make all these feelings and emotions a small problem. I wanted to magnify God in my life. I have always believed in God, or a supreme being. I look at the beauty that surrounds us in nature, and the human body. I am just amazed at the miracle of life. I have always believed very strongly that every situation in my life has happened for a reason. I just didn't always see the door open because I was standing in my shadow. I was not going to stand in my shadow this time and miss the door that God was going to open for me.

I tackled the darkness, the pain, the insecurities, and the unknown. Whenever I had a negative thought, I countered it with a positive thought. I'd wake up in the middle of the night with pain in my legs. I'd sit up and say, "Thank you, God, for letting me know that I am alive and that I have another day to enjoy!" God performs miracles and he displays his power among the people. It is through Him that we learn strength and courage. It is in the valleys that we grow! I placed my trust in God, knowing that He would carry me through this darkness. I would only see His '*Footprints*' in this time of trouble, not mine. He would carry me through it. "If God brought me to it, He will bring me through it."

Every morning I go outside just before sunrise, and with a positive affirmation, I celebrate the peace and love in my life with a joyous song in my heart. I close my eyes and use the following positive visualization.:

> *I take an even breath and listen*
> *to the glorious song of*
> *Creation all about me. I recognize*
> *that I am a perfect*
> *aspect of God's Divine plan. I*
> *allow myself to feel my*
> *connection to all life. I join in*
> *the celebration by adding*
> *my song to the music of the*
> *Universe. In my mind's eye*
> *I see myself going through my*
> *day in perfect harmony,*
> *Relating to all creation with*
> *peace and love. I combine*
> *these imagines with the feelings*
> *of joy and let them go,*
> *Knowing that they will create*
> *the good things I am*
> *Visualizing and thinking.*

As I sit and watch the miracle of the sun rising before me, I feel the warmth upon my face. I let go of all my worried thoughts and stress. I imagine an energy of light and love emanating from the sky that surrounds me with peace and a deep sense of relaxation. I see myself acting in a new way and accept this new me as real. I express thanks for two things in my life everyday!

We have a right to choose our thoughts. There is power in positive thinking. With positive thinking, we can make things happen. We start to enjoy being in love with life and living in harmony in our relationships. Health and energy comes to our bodies, success and prosperity in our financial affairs, and safety and protection is everywhere. It is a deep sense of peace when we are consciously connected to the Divine within ourselves. Your thoughts become your words and words are powerful. Words have the power to heal our wounds. They set up the vibrations of healing or illness within your body.

Positive affirmation reflects the way you want your life to be, not how it is today. Affirmations are a tool of creation. They reflect the spiritual law of perfection everywhere. They are based on spiritual truth. Affirmations are a positive statement of what you want your life to be. They are expressed in the present tense. For us, as patients with breast cancer, our affirmation is, "I am healthy and energetic. All of my cells are healthy and functioning perfectly." Marty Varnadoe Dow, LCSW has written a book, *Soar Above the Crisis*. It was recommended to me by one of the social workers who I worked with in the past. It is a wonderful book. It helped me understand who I am and provided techniques to help me *SOAR* above any crisis, and to stop struggling and start living!

Here are some positive affirmations that I found on the Internet at www. positivethoughts.com. It is a great web site with many resources available to you for free.

~I AM a good friend to myself and others.
~Today I fully experience the blessings that are all around me.
~Love is healing every aspect of my life. I AM whole and healthy.
~I have great respect for all the others who share my world.
~I AM a Divine being of light naturally expressing my life's purpose.
~I AM confident and optimistic that everything will unfold perfectly In my life.
~I embrace my fears with love and release them into the light.
~I easily and joyfully listen to my inner wisdom, always following its guidance.
~I expect good things to happen in my life because the Universe is supporting
        my success.
~I expect miracles for every person in my life.
~I claim my power. It is mine to use and I will use it well.
~I AM filled with gratitude and I expect to meet my blessings today.

~I accept my goodness in each and every moment of my day.
~I am speaking my truth today in love, knowing that it is valuable. I expect others to respect and value my opinions.
~I AM ready and willing to change for the better.
~Through the power of faith and trust I stay in the flow of God's goodness and mercy.
~Today I choose to think positive, loving and successful thoughts.
~I trust that my future is unfolding in perfect order. I expect my life to be filled with joy and success.
~I accept myself with love and I know that the doorway to greatness is opened before me. I walk through it with joy.
~I AM thankful for all the blessings in my life and all the blessings that are yet to come.
~My thoughts are powerful and therefore I choose them carefully.
~I choose joy and grace in my life.
~Today and everyday I AM standing in the power of love and everything in my life is flexible and flowing.
~I AM a positive thinker. This day and everyday my mind is filled with positive thoughts creating a beautiful and positive life for me.
~I accept myself, knowing that I am a work in progress. I recognize my potential as I love and honor my shortcomings.
~I have special qualities that only I bring to this world.
~I AM growing and changing easily at my perfect pace.
~I recognize my inner truth and I speak it easily and joyfully.
~Today, I choose to think only those thoughts that uplift and empower me.

These are powerful words to incorporate into your life, into your inner spiritual self, and your soul. Our souls are an ever-present part of our living being. We must nurture it, be kind and loving to it. Our souls are not something that ascends to the heavens when we pass from this life to another. It is who we are at this present moment.

I have placed these affirmations on small cards throughout our home. My husband thinks I'm silly but I have chosen to improve my life through positive thinking and affirmation, knowing that I am good and I am unique. I believe that to celebrate life, we have to share our own unique self with the world. What better way than through understanding ourselves and loving ourselves?

The power of visualization is easy to use. I have shared two or three visualizations with you earlier. Shakti Gawain stated, "*In order to use creative visualization to create what you want, you must be willing and able to accept the best that life has to your good."* What a concept! We use creative visualization every day and most of us don't even realize it. We have all daydreamed about an upcoming event, a new car, the perfect partner, mentally rehearsed an argument, the death of a loved one, or imagined the worst outcome to a situation that we were experiencing. Some people use mental images to create their positive visualizations, while others use words. The first step, however, is to determine what it is that you want to create in your life. If you are certain of the specific details of what you want to manifest in your life, clearly imagine those events in your mind's eye. For me, it was feeling healthy and full of energy again. I imagined every cell in my body free of illness and functioning normally.

In September, I will have a breast revision done. I am using positive visualization to create my new reality. I am going to have surgery, the incisions will heal well, and I will be pleased with the results of the revision. I will not be able to see or feel the implants. Another component is that my husband will no longer be fearful of hurting me when he touches my breast.

If you don't know the specifics of what it is that you want your life to be, or what you want in your life, then imagine a paint brush. You are making brush strokes on a canvas to define the general event or events in your life that you want, omitting the specific details. Then you have to patiently wait for God's force to fill in the details. Visualization is a powerful tool of the conscious mind. Combining visualization with prayer, faith, and love, you will be able to *soar* above the crisis you feel yourself, in this very moment, and any that will come your way.

Chapter Ten

Walk Hand In Hand

As we come to the end of our second year of this journey, I realized that we had put distance between us. It is as if we both have gone our separate ways. I spent so much time concentrating on surviving, and my husband spent his time concentrating on his career so that he didn't have to think about what had taken place. We had lost sight of "us."

We spent less time talking. We no longer laughed together. Our priorities changed. We no longer went to bed together, or had intimacy. It was as if we were two different and unconnected people, living under the same roof. The importance of family grew within me, and my ability to forgive those who had hurt me was beyond his comprehension. There were deaths in my family and I felt that I had to go to the memorial services for my ex-father-in-law. We had remained close and I had to do it out of respect for him and Mom.. I went to have closure, because my sons wanted and needed me to be there He was angry about it.

After some introspection, I realized that the past year had been all about me— the mastectomy, the chemotherapy and all the side effects. He had not traveled this journey with me hand-in-hand. He had not dealt with the life-threatening disease, other than to realize that he could have lost me to breast cancer. He did not go with me to my doctor's appointments, nor did he accompany me on the days that I had chemo-therapy. He had not shared my fear or my discomfort. Therefore, he could not understand, let alone comprehend, what a mastectomy does to your body imagine, your self-confidence and self-esteem. He didn't realize that part of the fight to survive is guilt and shame. I have to admit, that I did not realize that guilt and shame were part of it also, until several months ago. Oh, I probably did, but the words 'guilt' and 'shame' were not the words that I used, or even was aware of.

It came to a point near the holidays, that we needed to decide if our relationship was important enough to save. I felt that I was losing the partner that I waited twenty years for. I felt empty and alone, walking down a long, lonely, barren dirt road leading nowhere. I needed help.

Every night I would go to bed alone, crying, praying that God would open Wayne's heart and mine to the love that we had shared prior to this journey we had been forced to take. I wanted him to take my hand and walk with me, share the pain, the grief, and the loss of self that I had to rediscover myself. Wayne is forever telling me that I say the same things that his mother would say to him. I would pray that she would speak to him and open his heart, so he could understand what it is that he needs to do to help us rediscover us. I needed her help and God's, because whenever I told him what needed to occur, it never did. It was as if it landed on deaf ears. In his defense, I think that he did take this journey with me but he thought that if he didn't share his fears, stayed positive and maybe not even talk that I would feel better about all that had happened, and everything that I had felt.

I am not going to pretend that I have all the answers. I know that our marriage was based on love and respect, and we have had to fight through one of the toughest storms in the first fifteen months of marriage. If you asked me if it's worth saving, I would tell you yes, most definitely! It is not going to be easy. It will be another tough year of being patient, understanding, talking and listening, not reacting, and seeing a counselor. I am now ready to join a support group. I am going to strongly urge my husband to attend a group for spouses of breast cancer survivors. I married my husband with a strong commitment to our relationship. I did not marry him to fill a need. I love him very deeply and that is why I will make it work. I am the one with the power to save our marriage. Without telling him what I need, I can thank him for what he does do that makes me feel protected and safe, or remind him that laying in each others arms is the way it is supposed to be

I believe that we not only have to rediscover ourselves, who we are, and where this journey is taking us, but we have to rediscover our relationship with our spouses and significant others. Sometimes it is easier to just give up, but it does not make the road less difficult to travel. We can feel excited, content, peaceful, and happy.

I will spend the next year working at redeveloping our relationship. I know that the power is within me to achieve this. What is more important, I think, is that I want to save our relationship. Into another valley I will venture, learning what the Universe has to teach me, trusting in its power that everything will work out the way that it should. It may not happen as quickly as I would like, nor may it not turn out as I hope. Chances are it may turn out to be better than I ever expected or dreamed possible!

I know that you want to know all the details, and what happened to us. In time, I will be able to share that with you. For now, please be patient. I am traveling in the valley, to relearn. I am developing trust and understanding, and rekindling the fire of our love and devotion. We alone allowed this to happen to us. No one else, and no other thing caused this distance between us. We did it! It is up to "us" to take this journey, walking hand-in-hand, to rebuild and restore the gift that we were blessed with when we first met.

It is my hope that you will share my words of wisdom and every part of this journey with your spouse. He needs to be at the doctor's appointments with you. He needs to go to chemotherapy or radiation therapy with you. Together, both of you should look for support groups to attend separately. Keep your communication open, but don't react. Ask questions to find out exactly what both of you are feeling at the moment. Be honest with each other, and don't give up on closeness. You don't have to have sex, but you do need to be touched. Both of you do! Our spouses become the silent victim, and the forgotten survivor. As we fight to survive, we need to make sure that they are fighting to be a survivor as well. Otherwise, they become a victim and will never overcome the devastation of this journey. They will become lost to us, and our relationship will be lost. Hold on to him and take him along for the ride!

Chapter Eleven

Love Is Healing

To believe is to know that
Every day is a new Beginning.
It is to trust that Miracles happen,
And dreams really do come true.

To Believe is to see angels
Dancing among the clouds
To know the wonder of a stardust sky
And the Wisdom of the man in the moon.

To Believe is to know the
Value of a nurturing heart,
The innocence of a child's eyes
And the beauty of an aging hand,
For it is through their teachings we learn to love.

To Believe is to know we are not alone,
That life is a Gift and this
Is our time to Cherish it.

To Believe is to find the Strength
And Courage that lies within us.
When it is time to pick up
The pieces and begin again.

To Believe is to know the wonderful
Surprises that are just waiting to happen,
And all our Hopes and Dreams are within reach.

If only we Believe!

The reason I waited to have you read that poem is because the mind is powerful. Earlier, I spoke of being scared waiting for the results of the bone scan that my oncologist ordered. I spoke with Dr. Geoffrey and he reminded me that the mind is such great power. He told me that I needed to stay positive.

I think one of the biggest hurdles that we have after the treatment is over, is the fear of reoccurrence. The other is separation anxiety from those who have watched over us so closely during our treatment. We feel that we could camp out in the hall of their office building waiting to keep our appointments.

I believe that one of the things that we have to do, no matter how hard it may be for us, is to give our treatment credit. At the end of this initial journey, we have to stop and give ourselves credit for what we have achieved. We need to shift our gears into another phase in life, which is surveillance. What we have to remember is that we are still be watched…the intervals are just a little longer.

Being a breast cancer survivor is a marathon, not a sprint. We have to learn how to handle all the symptoms that will hang around after the treatments are done. We have to learn to make choices. We have to manage our expectations because the lingering effects of chemotherapy are going to be with us for awhile. We are going to feel fatigue and we will have to continue to have planned rest periods, and think about the part of the day and the activities that make us most tired. I have trouble finding words, or remembering names and places. I heard someone call that "chemobrain." I have to write things down, and ask people to repeat information. I have trouble staying focused with work, which is one of the most frustrating and troubling side effects I am having to deal with.

I have had to lower my expectations for myself so that I do not become frustrated, or lose my self-esteem, confidence, and self-worth. To do that, I needed help from my co-workers. I needed to let them know the problems I continued to have, and that I needed their help. We need to help others understand that we cannot jump back into doing all the things that we did before. We have to give up things that are less important to us, and work with the frustrating side effects.

I often ask myself if there ever will be a time when I don't worry about it coming back, or think about breast cancer. I honestly don't know. Some people say yes, but we are all different. I think the thought will recede like the tide, and there are entire days when I don't think about it. I find it difficult right now because I still see a different body in the mirror and it reminds me of what happened.

To believe, gives us hope and understanding that every day is a gift. To believe is to find the strength and courage that we have within ourselves to pick up the pieces and make new, and to begin again. You must trust in yourself, your treatment, and the knowledge of your physicians. You are worthy of a new start, and a new beginning. Our lives are like a train ride. Now we are back on the train experiencing a new world with all of our senses: taste, touch, smell, sight, listening and feeling. We can enjoy the extraordinary in the ordinary.

We did not take our honeymoon in 2002, when we were married because we wanted to go on an Alaskan cruise. We were waiting for the following summer. To our surprise, I was diagnosed with breast cancer in March, 2004, and our honeymoon had to be postponed. In 2005, it looked like we may not be able to take the cruise.

We made our arrangement for the cruise. We would fly to Vancouver, and then board the Holland Cruise line two days later. I have always wanted to go to Alaska. I love the mountains and the glaciers. I wanted to see the whales, to hear them sing, and I wanted to see the majestic mountains and absorb the history. I cannot wait to see the beauty, try different foods, and meet and talk to different people. I knew I would enjoy hiking up a trail in the fresh, mountainous air, while catching a glimpse of moose, bear, and elk. I wanted to see the beauty of the valleys, and the flowers that adorn them in all their wonder. I envisioned snow-capped mountains sitting above clear blue lakes.

As I think about taking the cruise, I realize that we will make new memories and begin a new passage of our life together. We will be able to bond once again, at a time that we are both healthy. Spiritually, we are growing and finding ourselves, and learning how to be at peace with ourselves.

As we fought to survive in our own way, I don't think he realized that he was fearful of hurting me, facing his own mortality, and feared losing me. If he was at work, then he didn't have time to think about what was actually happening. We grew apart. We were alienating each other. We started being critical of one another, and stopped being kind and considerate. As I told you previously, we stopped going to sleep together. When intimacy gets put on the shelf, you find yourself wondering where both of you have gone. What happened to 'us?' I found that I was reacting to what he said and his behaviors. As I look back, I think that the reaction is worse than the behavior itself. We did not argue. We just didn't talk.

This trip was going to be one of the most vital things we have done to re-discover us. Wayne is my soul mate and I will not lose him. I know the man that I married is still in there. We have not gone everywhere together during this past year. While I was concentrating on surviving and he on making a living, we forgot how to make a life. We will be married for three years in December, 2005, and I have made a commitment to resolve the strain that we have in our marriage. I know that happy marriages are not always happy. There will always be struggles, but with good communication, not reacting to behaviors and being positive, I can find the man that is nestled down within himself.

While on this cruise, it will just be us. There will be no stressors from work, or not working. We will relax, and find comfort in being with one another. As we become at peace internally, the kindness and gentleness will rise to the surface. I will reach for and hold his hand when we walk. We will honor one another once again.

The three days before we left, I spent time getting things ready. I cleaned the house, refrigerator, arranged pet sitting, went to the bank, and to the pet store for some treats while we were gone. I started laundry and pacing the day before. The excitement began to build, and we could not wait for the day to begin our new adventure. This would be the adventure of a lifetime because we would not only go sight-seeing, but we were going to rediscover the oneness we had lost.

We flew out of Phoenix on a Thursday morning and reached Vancouver early. We had our luggage taken to our room and then started walking down the streets of 'Old Vancouver.' There were tourist shops everywhere…shopping is an energy boost for me. I love to window-shop, but when I see something that really catches my eye, I buy it. Wayne has to go with me because he is the one who controls me and my shopping!

We bought a couple of gifts for our sons and their girlfriends. Then I saw the most beautiful Jade Butterfly necklace. Jade represents good luck and butterflies are symbolic of new life, so I just had to have it! It was so beautiful! For me, the butterfly was a symbol of our new life together, and the Jade would bring us luck.

We spent our first evening just walking around the city. In the morning, we planned to take a city tour. Our first stop was at 'Gas Town.' What a magical place. There were gaslights along the streets, large clocks on the corners and shops everywhere! We walked and shopped until we had to stop for lunch. We ate lunch in a quaint restaurant. We talked and I even got him to laugh by playing footsie with him! We didn't leave Gas Town until late in the afternoon and then picked up the tour bus again to go to Vancouver proper. The city was bustling with people working and shopping in the clothing and shoe stores. The residents live in apartment complexes which are skyscrapers. We inquired about the cost of the penthouses and they told us that they start at $250,000.00! An apartment there costs the same as an average home in Arizona! That was just amazing. the scenic view and the cooler summer weather, along with mild winters is something that some of us would like to experience if we have lived in the desert for awhile.

As we were finishing the tour, we stopped at a park along the beach. It was filled with lush trees and flowers. When I took a deep breath, I could smell the pine trees and the fragrance of flowers. Men and women would stop in a small flower shop in the park to buy fresh-picked flowers. We went through the second largest China Town in the country. If you have ever visited San Francisco, then experiencing Vancouver is just like it, only it's more beautiful because of the scenery, the mountains and the landscape.

We went to the port and went through customs. Then we boarded the ship. It was thrilling! The ship was like a small city. It was eloquently designed and the crew was so friendly and nice. Our stateroom was small but there was room to put everything away. We then decided to take a tour of the ship. There were shops, a casino, theaters, bars with live music, two pools, recreation room and several fine-dining restaurants.

There was so much to see out on the deck as the ship set sail for Alaska. The views were just breathtaking. As we entered the Inside Passage, we saw some humpback whales. Such magnificent creatures. Glacier Bay was one of the most amazing sites that we saw. The glaciers extended for miles wide and long. Imagine ice going into the depths of the ocean for a mile or more!

The most wonderful part of this trip, however, was walking around the deck with my husband. We held hands, and we felt the peace and contentment. I could feel the warmth and compassion starting to fill our souls once again. We were joining together as we had in our first year of marriage. We listened to one another, and we held one another. I could feel the love in our hearts growing, and building a bond that would not be broken. I was filled with an excitement...excited for the growth that we were now growing once again.

As we stopped at the small settlements, cities and the mountains stood with such pride. It was as if you could hear them speaking to you. Their wisdom and knowledge just filled your soul with peace and excitement! The clouds appeared to be sitting right on top of their peaks as if they were holding them up. The midst sitting in the firs was beckoning. Alaska is in the middle of a rain forest. It is much like Seattle, they told us, and that is why it is called the 'Land of the Rainbows.' We did see rainbows! You could follow them from the very beginning of their appearance, and when your eyes reached the end, it was illuminating! There was a bright light surrounding the end of the rainbow! That's the pot of gold I would guess.

The time just slipped away as we walked through Ketchikan, Skagway, and Juneau. I cannot begin to explain the beauty of the countryside. Even though it was raining and cold, it drew you close to nature and all the positive energy that it held. The air was so fresh and clean. It was invigorating! We found ourselves relaxed, able to share thoughts and moments of laughter. Wherever we walked, we held hands. There were times when Wayne would hold me tighter than normal, while we tried to get through a crowd of people, as if he was afraid that he would lose me.

We met a wonderful couple on the ship. We ate lunch with them towards the end of the cruise and I think that we sat there for a couple of hours. The men talked about their experiences in the service and us girls talked about Alaska and a little about our journey with breast cancer. They were both very interested in the metaphysical aspects of my experience. Although they were from Manhattan, they were very down-to-earth and simple people. They were enjoying their lives together. It was their second marriage, also. She had a friend who had been diagnosed with breast cancer and was very interested in reading *Surviving Breast Cancer: There Is A Child Within Us*. She will be participating in the Cancer Walk this fall.

We arrived home on a Sunday morning. For the next three days, we talked about our trip and our experiences in Alaska with each other, friends and family. Dreading to go back to work, the unpacking and cleaning made us even more exhausted than we already were! Sleep came easy with memories to last a lifetime. We were on our way to rediscovering us! It was going to be a slow process but one that would strengthen our loving bond, our companionship and friendship! This process will be difficult and it lies within my power to change our present relationship. I will be the one who will bring back the man that I married, and the person who I was. I am in control of the process that will either make our marriage strong or allow it to crumble. The mountain that I have had to climb is accepting the fact that I no longer am able to feel my husband's touch and enjoy the physical pleasure that it once gave me. I will have to learn to enjoy that we can be intimate without that pleasure. Just knowing that we are "together" is enough!

Faith is two empty hands held
open to receive all of the Lord."

-Alan Redpath

Reach high, for stars lie hidden
In our soul.
Dream deep, for every dream
Precedes a goal.

-Pamela Vault Starr

Chapter 11

Road To New Beginnings

Life is like a collage of beginnings and endings that seem to be like wet paint running together. Before we begin a new path on our journey, we have to find closure for the path we are leaving. I don't think we can understand the significance of an event in our life, until we do find closure. Finding closure opens the door for us to see the new path we will take on our journey of life and living.

It has been two years that I have been on this journey to rediscover myself. I've had to tie up the loose ends, and quiet my mind even if there were unanswered questions. For me, and I believe that for everyone, it acknowledges that a change has taken place. Finding closure allowed me to let go of my feelings, my fears, and my uncertainty, so I could honor the experience I had just been through. When I finally reached the point of closure, I was able to affirm I did what was needed to become a 'survivor' and developed wisdom for another path in my life's journey.

In our busy, noisy world, we find ourselves longing for peace and searching for a place somewhere else. I found that peace comes from within oneself. I learned to grow and cultivate peace within myself by realizing that I had to let my anxieties go. The details of my life would work themselves out without any guidance from me. I had to learn to let go, and to allow the power of the Universe to take hold, while trusting and believing that Devine intervention would take care of all my fear, worries and anxieties.

Deciding to find a means of inner peace was the first step. I learned to meditate on peace, and what it feels like to be calm and serene. It takes determination and a commitment to practice daily. Even throughout the day, when I started to feel myself getting anxious, I would take a break, breathing slowly and deeply. The clutter of thoughts In my mind would clear, and peace and serenity would fill my soul. With practice, my soul would hunger for those moments, and I realized I had the power to free myself from my own anxieties, worries and fears.

I have done a lot of reading these past two years. Something I have come to believe very strongly is we have the personal power within us to achieve our dreams and desires. I discovered this power and you can too. It enables you to be more sensitive, and it gives you a clear sense of strength. It creates an impact that we have on others. It is not overbearing or meek. Finding this inner power allowed me to feel my worth, and self-respect. It showed me I could work on behalf of my own dreams and desires. I had no reason to be ashamed or afraid.

Cheryl Richardson, in her book, *The Unmistakable Touch of Grace,* stated, "There are no coincidences. Every event we experience and every person we meet has been put in our path for a reason." In grace there is a creative force of exceptional kindness and goodness.

We have to surrender ourselves to let go of our fears, losses, and desires. We must allow our faith in the power of the Universe to take control. We have to learn to surrender before we allow ourselves to begin that path of suffering. Our soul doesn't control our life, our egos do. We have to give up our own will to find inner peace. Negative thinking prevents us from experiencing the positive power of the Universe—grace.

I know that I am repeating myself but I cannot stress the importance of finding inner peace. Bringing your mind to a state of silence through meditation heals the mind, rests the body, and opens your conscious to the remarkable awareness of your Soul—your spirit, which is intertwined and interconnected to all living things in the Universe. In my first book, I called this recognizing the Extraordinary in the Ordinary! This inner peace will help you have faith that all that is happening to you is the way it should be. Everything does happen for a reason.

In Daily Om, one of their articles compared the journey of water to our lives. We move through life encountering twists, turns, valleys and mountains just as a river meets with obstacles, twists and turns.

After reading this article, I had gone to one of my favorite places and sat beside a stream. I realized while watching the water that it is a great teacher! It moves with grace, ease and determination but with humility.

When we encounter the valleys in our lives coming down from the mountain, we fall hard but we keep on going. What the water teaches us is to be brave, not to waste time clinging to the past, and not looking back. It keeps moving forward because eventually it will reach a larger body of water. The water has no ego or fear of losing its identity or control.

When we allow ourselves to find inner peace, we become as a river. We move with grace, surrendering our past. We regain our identity. Grace touches our lives and we can move forward, letting go of our egos, and becoming part of something larger. Our personal lives expand and we are more aware of the beauty of nature, and we also realize we have a purpose in everyone's journey.

I started working at a home health company about a year ago. I struggled with this new territory. One day, I was at a meeting and our supervisor made the statement that, "We cannot achieve perfection, but we can achieve excellence."

What I realized was there is no such thing as perfection, especially in life. All of life is in a constant state of change and movement. Our lives are an experiment, helping us to experience and learn that we are imperfect. We are being reborn every day. Our hair grows, cells are constantly dying, and blood is continuously flowing.

I wanted, and I repeat, I wanted to be perfect for my husband. I wanted to go back to the way it was—the way our relationship was in the beginning of our marriage. I missed him and the closeness that we had shared. I wanted to look and feel the same—long white hair, tall and thin, full of energy, joy and happiness. That is the perfection that I remembered.

I was holding on or trying to force perfection and what I did not realize was that he was not, nor was anyone else, judging me to see if I was perfect. I remember talking to a friend and telling her I felt that I had a sign on my forehead that said I had breast cancer. I thought that anyone who looked at me could tell that I had a reconstructed breast and that my hair was a wig—or that the new growth was not the same as I had had before the chemotherapy. She smiled and asked me if I really thought that when people looked at me that they could really tell that I had had breast cancer and gone through chemotherapy? I sat there, then smiled and said no. I was forcing what I felt and what I saw when I looked into a mirror, onto them.

I realized that I could let go of the need to be perfect and experience the Universe as a loving place where I am free to be imperfect. It is humanly inherent to be imperfect. If I embraced my imperfections, I would be embracing myself! I had to broaden my sense of who I am, and learn to appreciate myself as a brave spirit on a mission—a mission of growth and becoming wise from the knowledge that I have learned on this journey of surviving breast cancer. Having had breast cancer does not mean the end. It is only the beginning of a new and wonderful life!

I had to teach myself to be patient and to tap into the wisdom I had learned on this journey to become a survivor. I needed to remember the bravery I had to

149

have in order to fight through all the challenges I have faced in my life. I had to learn to honor myself. In the movie, *"Tuesdays with Morrie,"* the professor told his former student, "You need to know how to die in order to know how to live." What a profound statement that holds so much wisdom. Working in hospice taught me that lesson. Teaching, supporting and understanding, and sharing experiences of their lives showed me that truly knowing how to die does teach those of us who survive, how to live. Death is a great teacher!

My fears became a barrier, but I realized, as noted in Chapter Four of this book, that the shortest distance through the darkness is running into it and not around it. Walking through my fears and facing them head-on would give me strength. Each time another fear appeared, I was able to stare that fear in the face, knowing the Universe would offer aid and support, thus finding faith in myself to grow.

Two years of emotional pain permeated my life. Pain is an act of being. Pain can become a shield which protects us from others, but in allowing this to happen, it gives us the identity of being a victim. I was determined to use that pain to be a survivor! I was not going to allow myself to become a victim. Being a survivor is a state of mind, one that is only dictated by the person going through the experience.

Pain is universal and it can and did empower me to use the hurt to help others. It allowed me and gave me the ability to help others with similar or different pain. I chose to transform that pain into healing love. The emotional pain helped me to draw energy from a pool of strength to emerge on the other side, and to pass that strength onto others. Helping others helped my own heart grow stronger, and it increased my feelings of self-worth and optimism. Reaching out to others declared to me that my pain did not defeat me. In fact, it helped me heal.

We must live in the moment. Each moment of our life is filled with richness and magic. Each second is a miracle and worthy of being savored. To live a balanced life, I have learned that we need to embrace the past, present and future simultaneously. Living in the moment allows us to appreciate all the beauty that is unique to that moment.

Our lives are so cluttered that we become overwhelmed by burdens, tasks, and responsibilities. Individual moments become lost. Each moment carries with it an immeasurable amount of pleasure and delight that we should not let pass without recognition and awareness. We need to be conscious of the present and its pleasures, and then let it go. When focusing on life's little pleasures, we relish everything we do, and we emerge fully in every experience, whether positive or negative. We need to learn to embrace the present and then we realize life's magnificence is its precious moments.

"Yesterday is the Past,
Tomorrow is the Future.
Today is the Present...
That is why it is called a Gift!
Use it wisely."

-Author Unknown

Chapter Twelve

Spiritual Path To Inner Peace

Being diagnosed with breast cancer, having a mastectomy, and going through chemotherapy was more devastating than I thought it would be. I am a nurse and I thought I would be able to handle it much better than I have. I also didn't realize that it would be so devastating to our marriage. Even though I thought myself to be strong, my world crashed. I found weaknesses that I didn't know that I possessed, and learned why I felt the way I did about my reactions, and my responses.

I was lost. I couldn't remember who I was, especially losing the happiness and joy that had filled my life for the two years prior. I was constantly fearful of what was coming next. I tried to stay in control but felt out of control. I felt I had lost myself, and my husband. I didn't recognize the person in the mirror's refection. I could not look at myself without crying and felt the very essence of my being disappear.

It has been three years and I still fight to be a survivor. Recently, I had shoulder surgery. While I sat on the gurney, an IV in my hand, and waiting for the surgeon, it brought back the day I was waiting for Dr. Geoffrey and Dr. Robert Leber to take me to surgery to remove my breast. I sat there and cried, literally sobbing. My husband, bless him, stood beside me and held me. He told me he understood and it was all right. It is all right! I will always cry, but I am okay!

The past several months have been extremely difficult. I found myself becoming what I had promised myself I would not allow—a victim! Instead of allowing others to dictate that state of mind, my very own thoughts were doing it. I was being negative, and had lost my self-confidence and esteem that I had gotten back. I was a lost soul once again, walking on a path without direction, and without a connection to anything or anyone.

I knew that I needed to find my way back. I had started a new job in the fall of 2005 with a home health company. I felt out of place and I did not feel that I had much value. I didn't feel that I was contributing to the success of the branch. I lost faith in my abilities to help caregivers provide good patient care. Oh, what a web I did weave. I became so depressed. I didn't smile, I couldn't sleep, and I was so tired I would cry. I read a quote from Helen Keller which changed the downhill course I was, "Life is a succession of lessons which must be lived to be understood." I sat down and thought about the lessons I thought I was supposed to learn and then wrote them down. I had to reach deeper within myself to understand why I felt, reacted, and was responding to these events in my life. I had to be honest, too. Honesty can be painful, but what a relief it can be. What a sense of inner peace it will bring when you can face the pain of why you are how you are.

No one is perfect. Life is not perfect. Life will only guarantee imperfection! When we are able to accept that, we are on the path to rediscovering ourselves. Cherie Carter-Scott, Ph.D., wrote in *If Life is a Game, These are the Rules,* she said that the real "you" is stored inside of this body—all hopes, dreams, fears, thoughts, expectations and beliefs that make each one of us unique. What I realized was my body was going to be with me for the duration of my life on earth. I could love it or hate it, accept it or reject it, but it was the only one I was going to get. I needed to change my relationship with my body. I knew the first step was to start back on the path to inner peace, contentment and happiness, and to make peace with my body. I was the one who had to make the decision of what to do next.

I know that I am repeating myself but write this down and keep it within sight: "Life does not guarantee perfection. It promises Imperfection." It is through imperfections that we learn from each experience. Isn't that what we are here for—to take this journey and learn from all of our experience and grow with wisdom? I had to make a choice between feeling worthless and unhappy or I could take some action and accept what had happened and make a positive change. The decision I needed to make was to let go of the former image I had of my body. I had to learn to treat by body as a temple of good, peace, and healing. I had to make time for myself, and allow my body to teach me pleasure through its five senses; sight, touch, smell, taste and hearing. I returned to enjoying the extraordinary in the ordinary that I spoke about in my first book. I learned to listen to my body.

When I got nervous or felt confused, I would close my eyes and start breathing slow and deep breaths so that I could relax. I concentrated on my breathing and would listen to each breath and I became surrounded by my nothingness. I could see the breaths flowing through every part of my body, and leaving behind it a sense of peace, serenity, and relaxation. I reminded myself,, my co-workers and those who had read my first book, *Surviving Breast Cancer – There Is A Child Within Us*, that this experience was a gift. It was not the end of life but only the beginning. Every experience and circumstance that I have faced and will face is an opportunity to learn, and find inner peace. Through introspection and meditation, came understanding of how to make a choice. It is done by your very essence—your soul connected to the "Universe." I had to start at the very beginning of my beliefs.

Everything happens for a reason, which is part of a Devine intervention. It leads us on a unique path, and presents us with special gifts. As we live in each moment through our trials and tribulations, successes and failures help us develop a unique wisdom which is ours alone. When we share our stories, we not only heal ourselves but we let others know that they are not alone. We help each other by listening and sharing, without judgment. I don't have any secrets, and I am not telling you that this is an easy process. It is a painful process because you have to face events, or words that have hurt you, either emotionally or physically. The deeper I looked inside, the more I recalled my childhood and young adulthood experiences. They were painful, and influenced my behavior, however, they now affected my feelings and reactions in the present.

All the answers that I was looking for were already within my grasp. All I needed to do was look inside, listen, believe and trust myself. I needed to take responsibility for the way I was feeling and then catapult myself into changing my life! Our life, and our reactions to life's lessons, are the only thing we can control. I looked up the Serenity Prayer and typed it on several pieces of paper which I have placed in various places at home and at work:

> *Grant me the Serenity to accept*
> *The things I cannot change,*
> *The courage to change the things I can,*
> *And the Wisdom to know the difference.*

I read this prayer every time I am faced with making a decision or when I have heard something that causes me anxiety. I also read it when I have made a mistake which makes me feel bad. I sit back and think, "What can I learn from this?" Can I change something? If not, I take a deep breath and just "let it be." If I can make a change, then I determine the best course of action with love and compassion.

No one has a perfect life. We have choices. We have to accept ourselves as we are, where we have been, and where we are in the present. It is the only way we can become comfortable with ourselves. It is no coincidence that someone enters our life. We don't have to understand why our paths have joined. If we allow ourselves to believe there are no accidents, then no coincidences can give up our confusion, our fear, anticipation, resentment, and our resistance. We can be filled with gratitude for every experience, and everything we have for those things we do not have. Being grateful is a choice which empowers us to change our perspective on every circumstance we face in our lives.

The most recent lesson I have learned is understanding why I now work in home health. I was guided down this path so that I could join with my present co-workers, one in particular, Linda, because I needed to re-learn (to be shown) that I have value as a person, as a nurse, and as a manager in the company, and to myself as a human being. It has taken a year, but I have achieved a sense of gratitude for where I am in life, because it is where I am meant to be.

There is power in the four words, *"I am a Survivor."* We will all walk this path in our own personal way, and recovering at our own pace, with the methods that we are most comfortable with. When we become grateful for who we are, with our bodies, where we are at in life, then we become empowered to make changes in the way we view life and the good and bad trips that it takes us on. We are spirits from the moment of conception. We occupy a body to travel our life's journey. We learn the lessons that we are meant to learn, and we become wise until we have achieved our purpose in life and pass on to another life.

Let go of the pain and rejoice, laugh, love, share, and listen to others so your soul will be filled with peace. Allow yourself to travel through life gracefully. Enjoy the extra-ordinary in the ordinary, connecting with the positive energy of the Universe. Allow it to flow freely throughout your body, heart, mind and soul. Remember always—*Having breast cancer is not the end of life. It is just the beginning!*

Chapter Thirteen

Food For Thought

As I re-read through pages of notes that I have made over the past year, I came upon quotes that I had written down. Under some of those, I made notes. It appeared that certain words touched my soul. I had meditated on what those quotes had said to me, and as I thought back to when I wrote them, they were teaching me wisdom and giving me strength.

Being diagnosed with breast cancer, or any life-threatening disease, causes a crisis. It is painful, frightening, and a difficult path. There will always be a crisis in our lives. These trials are not something that we ask for, but I now believe that they can be an adventure of a lifetime! We cannot sit in sad remembrance of days gone by, nor curse what has happened to us while hanging our heads and crying. We have to look forward to what life holds for us. I want to feel the winds of change blowing in my face.

I want to see what life is going to unfold for me. How about you? I want to see what's coming up, and not look at the past. Life's too short for yesterdays. It moves along too fast. So when our ride gets bumpy, when we look back, we need to look up front and see if our life will jump the track. It is all right to remember this part of our history, but what's in front of us is where it is happening. The enjoyment of living is not where we have been. Rather, it is looking ever forward to another year.

Crisis is a double-edged sword. The diagnosis of breast cancer brings the destruction of life as we have known it. It threatens our egos, and it creates chaos where there was stability. It will challenge our beliefs and response patterns. This crisis places us in an emotional turmoil and we lose the ability to cope. Breast cancer also brings with it the opportunity for something new to develop from the ruins it has created in our OLD way of life!

This crisis offers many hidden benefits to those of us who accept the adventure to transform ourselves in the face of this devastating event in our life and the lives of our loved ones. It gives us the opportunity to change directions and make important changes in our life. It is through this time that most of us learn the meaning of life. We discover our mission, which will give us a greater sense of direction and purpose.

We find our inner strength that we did not know existed. Some of us will tap into the inner guidance that I spoke of for direction. We re-evaluate beliefs that have negatively impacted our life experiences.

This life-threatening disease invites us to experience and release old fears. Many people will find, as I did, a deeper co-existence with God or the creative force in the Universe. For some, they may develop a profound sense of trust, knowing there is someone or something other than themselves that is watching over us.

Being diagnosed with breast cancer was an opportunity for me, not a certainty. I chose to take advantage of the energy in this crisis. I decided not to surrender to the feelings of despair and hopelessness. The adventure began when I CHOSE to accept the challenge and to use this life-altering circumstance as a stepping stone into a journey that was by far greater than I could have ever imagined.

I have documented a collection of quotes that have come to mean a great deal to me in this fight to be a breast cancer survivor, and to rediscover who I am, and where this journey is taking me. I hope that when you read through these quotes, if only one of them moves you, that you will write it down on a piece of paper. You need not think deeply, but write down why it moved you. It will become a source of strength for you. I hope that you enjoy them!

"All seasons are beautiful for the person who carries happiness within." ~ Horace Friess

"Listen to the Exhortation of the Dawn!

> Look to this Day!
> For it is Life, the very Life of Life.
> In its brief course life
> All the verities and Realities of your Existence.
> The Bliss of Growth,
> The Glory of Action,
> The Splendor of Beauty;
> For Yesterday is but a Dream,
> And Tomorrow is only a Vision;
> But Today well lived
> Makes every yesterday a Dream of Happiness,
> And every Tomorrow a Vision of Hope.
> Look well therefore to this Day!
> Such is the Salutation of the Dawn!" ~ Kalidasa

"Happiness is not so much in having as sharing. We make a living by what we get, but we make a life by what we give." ~Norman MacEwan

"I do not want a peace that passeth understanding. I want the understanding which bringeth peace." ~Helen Keller

"The beginning of wisdom is found in doubting; by doubting we come to the question, and by seeking we may come upon the truth." ~Pierre Abelard

> "One ship sails East,
> And another West,
> By the self-same winds that blow,
> 'Tis the set of the sails
> And not the gales,
> That tells the way we go.
>
> Like the winds of the sea
> Are the waves of time,
> As we journey along through life,
> 'Tis the set of the soul,
> That determines the goal,
> And knows the calm or the strife." ~Ella Wheeler Wilcox

"In the depth of winter, I finally learned that there was within me an invincible summer." ~Albert Camus

"Character cannot be developed in ease and quiet. Only through experience of trial and suffering can the soul be strengthened, vision cleared, ambition inspired, and success achieved." ~ Helen Keller

~Wisdom is the art of coping with suffering, it has its beginning in the willingness to tackle it head-on.

"Slow yourself down. Take one experience at a time. Savor those experiences and feelings in the very moment that you are experiencing them. While you are noticing them, be grateful for the person that you are, for who you are becoming, and for the experiences that you have.

"To live happily is an inward power of the soul." ~Marcus Aurelius

"Slow down and enjoy life. It's not only the scenery you miss by going too fast, you also miss the sense of where you are going and why." ~ Eddie Cantor

"Happiness is a journey, not a destination; happiness is to be found along the way, not at the end of the road, for then the journey is over and it's too late. The time for happiness is today, not tomorrow." ~Paul H. Dunn

"Most of the shadows of this life are caused by standing in one's own sunshine." ~Ralph Waldo Emerson

"There is only one way to happiness and that is to cease worrying about things which are beyond the power of our will." ~Epicteus

"Sadness is but a wall between two gardens." ~Kahlil Gibran

"Whether you're a candle in a corner, or a beacon on a hill, let your light shine brightly." ~Anonymous

"At the timberline where the storms strike with the most fury, the sturdiest of trees are found." ~Hudson newsletter

"When one door closes, another opens. But we often look so regretfully upon the closed door that we don't see the one that has opened for us." ~Alexander Graham Bell

"The best way to celebrate life is to share your own unique self with the world."

"In every life, there is a purpose. In every journey, there is meaning."

"You find strength, courage and confidence by every experience in which you really stop to look fear in the face. You are able to say to yourself, "I have lived through this...I can take the next thing that comes along. You must do the thing you think you cannot do." ~Eleanor Roosevelt

"I'd like to do everything I can to avoid being an old person who says, Why didn't I do that? Why didn't I take that chance?" ~Barbra Streisand

"It is in men, as in soils, where sometimes there is a vein of gold which the owner knows not of." ~Jonathan Swift

"When you encounter difficulties and contradictions, do not try to break them, but bend them with gentleness and time." ~St. Francis de Sales

"Be willing to have it so. Acceptance of what has happened is the first step to overcoming the consequences of any misfortune." ~William James

"God does not take away trials or carry us over them, but strengthens us through them." ~E.B. Pusey

"Your presence is a present to the world. You're unique and one of a kind. Your life can be what you want it to be. Take the days just one at a time. Don't put limits on yourself. So many dreams are waiting to be realized. Decisions are too important to leave to chance. Reach for your peak, your goal, your prize. Nothing wastes more energy than worrying. The longer one carries a problem, the heavier it gets. Don't take things too seriously. Live a life of serenity, not a life of regrets. Count your blessings, not your troubles. You'll make it through whatever comes along. Within you are so many answers. Understand, have courage, be strong." ~Douglas Pagels

"Happy the man and happy he alone, He who is secure within can say, "Tomorrow doesn't matter, for I have lived today." ~Horace

"Happiness is the grace of being permitted to unfold...all the spiritual powers planted within us." ~Franz Werfel

"If we are ever to enjoy life, now is the time. Today should always be our most wonderful day." ~Thomas Dreier

"To live is not merely to breathe, it is to act; it is to make use of our organs, senses, faculties, of all those parts of ourselves which give us the feeling of existence. The man who has lived longest is not he man who has counted most years, but he who has enjoyed life most." ~Jean-Jacques Rousseau

"I find ecstasy in living; the mere sense of living is joy enough." ~Emily Dickenson

"Happiness is neither within us only, nor without us; it is the union of ourselves with God." ~Blaise Pascal

"The rest of your life can be the Best, if you live with Purpose today. ~Author unknown

"Happiness is…the grace of being permitted to unfold…
all the spiritual powers planted within us." ~Franz Wefel

"Your presence is a present to the world. You're unique and one of a kind. Your life can be what you want it to be. Take the days just one at a time. ~Author unknown

"Come…let us take courage, and hand-in-hand pursue our journey in the path of life." ~Thomas A. Kempis

"Be willing to have it so. Acceptance of what has happened is the first step to overcoming the consequences of any misfortune." ~William James

"Life demands from you the strength you possess." ~Dag Hammarskjold

"Whatever came to me, I looked on as God's gift for some special purpose. If it was a difficulty, I knew He gave it to me to struggle with, to strengthen my mind and my faith." ~Author unknown

"…beginning today and lasting a lifetime through—hang in there, and don't be afraid to feel like the morning sun is shining…just for you!" ~Douglas Pagels

"I expect my life to be good and joyous, and it is! ~ Author unknown

"I create new memories filled with peace, goodwill, and compassion for others. ~Author unknown

"I trust in the Power that created me to protect me at all times and under all circumstances. ~Author unknown

"Problems test our character and our abilities. Obstacles challenge us to think creatively and figure out how to go under, over, around, or through them on our way to our goals. When the odds are against us, that is when we rise to the occasion and surprise people…including ourselves!" ~Author unknown.

"People are like stained-glass windows. They sparkle and shine when the sun is out, but when the darkness sets in, their true beauty is revealed only of a light from within." ~Elizabeth Kubler-Ross

"No one knows the mysteries of life or its ultimate meaning, but for those who are willing to believe in their dreams and in themselves, life is a precious gift in which anything is possible." ~Dena Dilaconi

Count your blessing, not your troubles. You'll make it through whatever comes along. Within you are so many answers. Understand, have courage, be strong. ~Author unknown

Find Happiness in Everything You Do

> "Find happiness in nature
> In the beauty of a mountain
> In the serenity of the sea
> Find happiness in friendship
> In the fun of doing things together
> In the sharing and understanding
> Find happiness in your family
> In the stability of knowing
> That someone cares
> In the strength of love and honesty
> Find happiness in yourself
> In your mind and body
> In your values and achievements
> Find happiness in everything
> You do." ~Susan Polis Schutz

"Feeling of anger, bitterness, and hate are negative. If I kept them inside of me they would spoil my body and my health. They are of no use." ~Dalai Lama

"A bend in the road is not the end...unless you fail to make the turn." ~Author unknown

"Don't stand in someone else's shadow when it's your sunlight that should lead the way." ~Author unknown

"Appreciate yourself by allowing yourself the opportunities to grow, develop, and feel a sense of purpose in this life." ~Author unknown

Thank You for allowing me to share my journey with you. The fight to be a survivor is difficult. It is a marathon. We have to re-learn, rediscover who we are, and be open to where our journey will take us. There are many battles that we face as we go through surgery and treatment, dealing with loses. Each of us feels differently about those loses; our breasts, losing our hair, loss of energy, pain and suffering. We struggle to regain our self-confidence and self-esteem.

We each cope with these in our own unique, and individual way. We learn something about ourselves on this journey. We have a resolve, and a strength that we did not know that we had within us. We learn that life is too short for yesterdays. We jump on the train, out front, so that we can feel the winds of change blowing in our faces so we can see what life unfolds for us! We learn that enjoyment of living is not where we have been, but where we are going.

One lesson that I have learned is that I had to allow myself to grieve. I could not allow the practical, medical side of me to stay at the surface. I had to allow myself to be a woman, a mother, a wife and let all the feelings that I had surface. I had to feel the emptiness, feel alone, feel the fear of what was going to be, fear I could not work with hospice patients, fear of losing my husband's affection. I had to feel lost and overwhelmed with anxiety. I had to allow myself to become angry with my new body image, and the loss of my desire to be intimate with my husband in order to find the appropriate path to rediscover myself. I had to stop setting expectations that my body could not meet.

There are many times that we have to allow others to suggest what may be wrong which forces us to think. With soul-searching we then find the source of our insecurity, our low self-confidence, and self-esteem. We are happy to be alive and breathing, but it is shadowed by a cloud of heaviness in ourselves. We have to take baby steps forward into this new life. We are children growing once again, depending on our family, friends, doctors, and co-workers for understanding and support.

Being a survivor is a difficult journey with a multitude of paths that we must take, but they are ours to take! We decide what path, during the course of this journey, is best for us. Others within our circle of family and friends will have to follow with us. We cannot, and you must not, allow others to place their opinions on you. They are theirs alone. The fight to be a survivor will be a life-long commitment. There will be other valleys that we must enter, and other mountains that we must climb.

However, this present journey will have given us the strength, courage and resolve to walk straight into the fear of the unknown and conquer it! We have learned that in the face our fear and darkness, the quickest path to the light which we seek, although the most difficult, is to walk directly into it.

There is no wrong or right path. It is the path that you have chosen for yourself that allows you to find that inner burning fire to survive. Normal is no longer in existence! Learning to enjoy yourself, your family and friends, and allowing the Universe to take care of itself will bring the inner peace and tranquility that we have searched for in the face of this life-threatening disease.

I learned that sometimes I just had to take one moment at a time, then one hour, and then a day. Through this method, I was enabled to have more good days than bad ones. It felt so good to be able to smile and laugh again. I was gradually able to accept all that had happened and be thankful that I was alive, and still full of life! There is nothing more important than health, family and happiness!

Enjoy life! See the extraordinary in the ordinary. Being diagnosed with breast cancer does close the door to your life as you once knew it. Do not allow the shadow to keep you from seeing the door which has now opened to you. Life is a gift! **Make each and every day the *Best Day* of your life. *Dance* as if no one is watching. *Sing* as if no one can hear.**

Find strength and courage in your family and friends. Be a friend to yourself! Do not allow others to place their feelings or opinions on you. Accept them as theirs alone. Survivorship is a state of mind dictated by you and you alone. You become a victim when you allow others to tell you how you should feel, when you should talk, and when you should cry. We will always cry about our loss.

The 'cancer worry' will always ebb with the tide every time we get sick. That is normal! You will find your own path on this journey, which will allow you to heal. Do not set expectations of yourself that you cannot reach. Just take one day at a time! If that is too much, then take one hour at a time.

This journey is about you re-learning, developing, and rediscovering yourself. No one can tell you how to do it, how long it should take, or how you should feel. This is your journey. As it is mine! I still have an occasional bad day. When I am feeling bad, I take a few minutes to breathe deep. I close my eyes and find my 'safe place' for comfort and peace. I sink deep into myself and allow the love and positive energy that surrounds me to flow within. I bring the peace and comfort back with me so that I can go on for the next hour, and the next, and the next, until it is tomorrow. What lies ahead of me is far too important to let slip away because I have been fretting about the yesterdays. The present is what is important. It is a gift, so use it wisely!

Celebrate life and living! *Share your unique self with the world.* There is a purpose to every life, and in every journey we take, there is meaning and reason. Happiness comes from within us. If we allow the positive energy within—our spiritual self, to connect to that which surrounds us—the wonder of nature, we will be filled with peace. Don't waste time worrying about things. You will discover a sense of direction and purpose, peace and serenity. Release your fears and then realize what an experience life and living will become! *You can transform your life in the face of this crisis. Remember that CAN, is the beginning of the word, "cancer!"*

As survivors, we have a destiny. We are not alone. We have come together to make Breast Cancer Awareness a reality to discovering prevention and cure. Stand tall! Be strong! Stand up and shout, "I'm a Survivor!" Those four words have such power and strength! Be proud! Each day is a gift.

I am very thankful to share my journey with so many wonderful men and women. I have been chosen to participate in this re-awakening. You have blessed my life in so many ways. God's angels of healing will be with you and they will surround you with their white light of love and protection. God Bless!

Debbie Ziemann, R.N., Breast Cancer Survivor

A Tear-Stained Life

Everything you seek in life
Everything you attain
Will be acquired through some tears
A lot will fall like rain.

All the happiness that you seek
All that you pray for
The tears will always come to you.
Like a storm, they will always pour.

The joy that you continually seek
The joy for which you pray
Is with you everyday of your life.
Your tears will show you the way.

The love that everyone hopes to find
The love that is meant for you
Always contains a lake of tears.
Your tears know when a love is true.

All this and more is in each tear.
Happiness, joy, love, and pain
Look back upon your life so far
You'll see that it is tear-stained.

-Chee Chee Martin, 2005

Suggested Readings

Bayda, Ezra with Bartok, Josh. *Saying Yes To Life (Even the Hard Parts)*, Boston, Wisdom Publications, 2005.

Casey, Karen. *Change Your Mind and Your Life Will Follow*. Boston,: Conari Press, 2005.

Chopra, Deepak. *The Book of Secrets, Unlocking The Hidden Dimensions of Your Life*. New York, Three Rivers Press, 2004.

Journey Into Healing, Awakening The Wisdom Within You. New York, Three Rivers Press, 1994.

Hanh, Thich Nhat. *Taming the Tiger Within, Meditations on Transforming Difficult Emotions New York:* Riverhead Books, 2004.

Cheryl Richardson, The Unmistakable Touch of Grace, New York, New York Free Press, 2005

Eleanor Wiley with Caroline Pincus, There Are No Mistakes, York Beach, ME, Conari Press,2006

Pollan, Stephan M., and Levine, Mark. *It's All In Your Head, Thinking Your Way to Happiness*. New York: Harper Collins Publishers, 2005.

Price, John Randolph. *The Angels Within Us*. New York,Ballantine Books,1993.

It's All In Your Head, Thinking Your Way to Happiness; Stephan M. Pollan and Mark Levine, Harper Collins Publishers, 2005

*Saying Yes To Life (Even the Hard Parts),*Ezra Bayda with Josh BartokWisdom Publications, 2005

Ryan, M.J. *The Happiness Makeover (How To Teach Yourself To Be Happy And Enjoy Every Day)*Broadway Books, 2005.

Recommended Web Sites:

www.BenefitLife.com

www.DailyOM.com

www.MartyDow-PositiveThoughts.com

Endorsement

Her experience as a caregiver in every aspect of her life has provided Debbie with the confidence and encouragement to be the survivor she describes in her writing. I have known Debbie both professionally and personally for six years. Her ability to persevere each day comes from the deep devotion she has in recognizing the great wonders of our imagination, and the confidence that a greater being provides us not only with the challenges of life, but gives us the tools to survive.

Persons of all ages and walks of life will gain confidence that they too can master their challenges as they read this true survivor's writing of the struggles of breast cancer and the demands those struggles place on each individual she has contact with, particularly her husband and children.

............Patricia Stock, R.N., and friend

Debbie writes in a candid manner that is both refreshing and insightful. She tackles subjects that other authors skirt around or never even mention. The result is a book which helps and encourages survivors of breast cancer in many ways and on multiple levels.

............Sabra House, LCSW, Psychotherapist, The Lighthouse Center.